Praise for *Unexpected Recoveries*

"Sensible, informative, and well written"

"Over the past twenty-five years, health writer Tom Monte has helped many leading figures of natural medicine tell their stories. When you see Tom Monte's name on a book, you know it will be sensible, informative, and well written. Now, with *Unexpected Recoveries,* Monte has entered a new dimension. He proves himself to be not just a medical writer but a medical philosopher of the first order. If you are suffering from an intractable illness such as cancer, you must read this book. It goes beyond the usual welter of pills, potions, remedies, and diets to an understanding of the principles of health."

–Ralph W. Moss
Author of the best-selling books
The Cancer Syndrome and *The Cancer Industry*

OTHER BOOKS BY TOM MONTE

The Complete Guide to Natural Healing

Controlling Crohn's Disease the Natural Way
(with Virginia Harper)

Freedom from Disease
(with Peter Morgan Kash and Jay Lombard, DO)

Living Well Naturally (with Anthony J. Sattilaro, MD)

Natural Prozac (with Dr. Joel Robertson)

Peak-Performance Living (with Dr. Joel Robertson)

Pritikin: The Man Who Healed America's Heart
with Ilene Pritikin)

Recalled by Life (with Anthony J. Sattilaro, MD)

Stop Inflammation Now! (with Richard M. Fleming, MD)

Taking Woodstock (with Eliot Tiber)

The Touch of Healing (with Alice Burmeister)

The Way of Hope

When Hope Never Dies (with Marlene McKenna)

World Medicine

UNEXPECTED RECOVERIES

SEVEN STEPS TO HEALING
BODY, MIND & SOUL WHEN
SERIOUS ILLNESS STRIKES

TOM MONTE

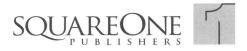
SQUAREONE
PUBLISHERS

The information and advice contained in this book are based upon the research and the personal and professional experiences of the author. They are not intended as a substitute for consulting with a health care professional. The publisher and author are not responsible for any adverse effects or consequences resulting from the use of any of the suggestions, preparations, or procedures discussed in this book. All matters pertaining to your physical health should be supervised by a health care professional. It is a sign of wisdom, not cowardice, to seek a second or third opinion.

COVER DESIGNER: Jeannie Tudor
TYPESETTER: Gary A. Rosenberg

Square One Publishers
115 Herricks Road | Garden City Park, NY 11040
516-535-2010 | 877-900-BOOK | www.squareonepublishers.com

Library of Congress Cataloging-in-Publication Data

Names: Monte, Tom, author.
Title: Unexpected recoveries : seven steps to healing body, mind, and soul when serious illness strikes / Tom Monte.
Description: Second edition. | Garden City Park, NY : Square One Publishers, [2017] | Includes bibliographical references and index.
Identifiers: LCCN 2016043898 (print) | LCCN 2016044487 (ebook) | ISBN 9780757004001 (pbk. : alk. paper) | ISBN 9780757054006
Subjects: LCSH: Catastrophic illness. | Sick—Psychology. | Terminally ill. | Chronically ill. | Healing.
Classification: LCC R726.8 .M665 2017 (print) | LCC R726.8 (ebook) | DDC 616.02/9—dc23
LC record available at https://lccn.loc.gov/2016043898

10   9   8   7   6   5   4   3   2   1

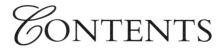

CONTENTS

PUTTING IT ALL TOGETHER

CONCLUSION

*To Toby, the foundation
of all that has been good.*

ACKNOWLEDGMENTS

This book is the culmination of more than thirty years of writing about health and healing. Although it would be impossible to thank all the people who contributed to my understanding of these infinite mysteries, I would like to mention a handful of individuals.

I would like to express my overflowing gratitude to my great mentors, Michio and Aveline Kushi, and Nathan and Ilene Pritikin, who gave me a foundation for understanding health and healing from both the Eastern and Western perspectives. Still under-appreciated, these four great teachers have provided countless millions of people with a path for better health and personal transformation.

I would like to thank some of my friends and teachers who have contributed to my work over the years, including Luc DeCuyper, Denny Waxman, Michael Rossoff, Bill Tims, Robert Pritikin, Mary Burmeister, Herman and Cornelia Aihara, Wim Mestdagh, John McDougall, Michael Jacobson, and Anthony Sattilaro.

My gratitude goes out to the many hundreds of people who have shared their stories of recovery with me over the past thirty-plus years, and the healers with whom I have worked. Not all of you appear in this book, but all of you contributed to it.

My sincerest thanks go out to Ken and Sherry Courage, Peter and Maryla Wallace, and Phiya Kushi, who also supported this work.

I would like to thank my wonderful friend and publisher, Rudy Shur; my editor, Michael Weatherhead; and the rest of the team at Square One Publishers for their tremendous talent, dedication, and commitment to releasing this book.

Finally, I would like to thank my wife, Toby, who wrote the recipes and menus for this book, and who has acted as the foundation of health and happiness for me and our entire family for forty years.

A NOTE TO CAREGIVERS

Each of us is plunged into his or her own private crisis whenever a loved one or dear friend is stricken with a serious illness. Driven by love, fear, and an overwhelming desire to help, caregivers will often spring into action, forgetting their own needs and limitations. Despite the best of intentions, a caregiver's self-sacrifice can to lead to exhaustion, anger, and conflict—not to mention poor health.

If you are a caregiver to someone who is ill, please consider adopting your own version of the seven steps described in this book. They can help you find rest so that you may have the strength to live more fully; care so that you can go on providing care; love so that you can go on loving; faith so that you can sustain hope; and strength of purpose so that you can find meaning in the challenges you are facing. Giving cannot be sustained without balance, meaning that those who give must also receive, and those who serve must also be served. Balance is the foundation of health and the consequence of love.

Please consider participating with your loved one as he or she utilizes the seven steps to restore his or her health by adopting your own version of this healing program. The program can be yet another act of love—a gift you give to your loved one as well as to yourself.

$\mathcal{J}$NTRODUCTION

eople overcome the most devastating diseases. Choose any illness that is now considered incurable and with a little effort you will find someone who has accomplished the unexpected feat of defeating that disease. Over the past thirty-five years, I have written about many hundreds of people who conquered illnesses that had been diagnosed as life-threatening or even terminal by medical doctors. In most of these cases, conventional medicine had run out of answers. In others, doctors had urged their patients to adopt some form of experimental treatment that, in fact, offered little hope of recovery. Yet these people overcame their illnesses and restored themselves to good health.

I have found that those people who were able to beat their diagnoses tended to follow a similar healing path, one with seven common steps. They were able to:

- get past their fears and establish more compassionate relationships with themselves.
- take back their power, in large part by taking responsibility for decision-making in their own recoveries.
- adopt a healing diet composed largely of plant food.
- establish a strong support system that included loving relationships, social support groups, and healers.
- make a commitment to life and to their healing programs.
- develop faith, which can be strengthened through various forms of spiritual practice, especially through daily prayer and meditation.
- find a purpose for living that transcended mere survival.

The intention of this book is to offer an action plan for the use of complementary healing methods, which can be used in conjunction with traditional medical treatment. In the chapters that follow, each healing step is described in detail, and practical guidance is provided to show you how to incorporate each step into your life.

The complementary modalities described in this book are supported by scientific literature, which is cited throughout the text. These are not simply "alternative practices." They are powerful healing tools whose degrees of effectiveness have been demonstrated both through human experience and in scientific studies.

The seven steps detailed in the following pages form an integrated, holistic program. Every step is important—indeed essential—but the foundation of this healing program is a plant-based diet, as step three makes clear. There are many expert and well-known practitioners of plant-based diets today, and I have provided contact information for several of them in the Resources. (See page 217.) Rather than provide personal case histories for each of these different programs, I have chosen to illustrate the seven steps with stories of the macrobiotic diet and lifestyle or the Pritikin program in particular. These are two of the oldest, most widely adopted, and most closely studied approaches to healing found in the world today. Both beautifully demonstrate the powers of a plant-based diet to restore health, even in people considered extremely ill. And as you will see, the scientific support for adopting a plant-based diet—including in the treatment of serious illness—is overwhelming.

Suggestions for how to incorporate this seven-step program into your daily life are provided in the closing chapters of this book, while recipes and a weekly menu plan may be found in the Recipes section. (See page 181.)

The potency of these seven steps depends to a great extent on the spirit of the person using them. A sincere commitment to getting well is fundamental to the healing process, and no one step has as much power to heal as when all seven are followed. As with so many other experiences in life, this is another case in which the whole is greater than the sum of its parts.

I have stressed throughout this book that people who use these methods should remain under the supervision of their doctors. As you incorporate the seven steps, your doctor can monitor you, inform you of any changes in your condition, and advise you in your medical choices. While it is important to remain in contact with your physician, it is essential that you explore other sources of information and become fully engaged in your own healing process. Only in this way may you fully utilize the healing powers within yourself, which, I am sure you will see, are far more powerful you think.

GET PAST THE SHOCK

This is how it starts. A medical doctor discovers the presence of a life-threatening illness for which there is only a slim chance of recovery or no medical solution at all—the inescapable message being that you are not likely to live much longer. Although your loved ones gather around you and offer their support, there is no one who really understands your situation or how alone you feel.

As remarkable as it may seem, an untold number of people find a way back to health after having been confronted with precisely this news. Through a series of experiences, some of which they initiate and others that appear unexpectedly, they discover healing tools, transform their lives, and overcome their diseases.

Marlene McKenna was one of these people.

When Marlene was thirty-eight years old, she discovered a growth on her back that was clearly suspicious. The growth was removed and biopsied. The diagnosis was unequivocal: Clark's level III melanoma, which meant that the cancer was malignant and had perhaps even spread. Surgeons removed the lymph nodes surrounding the tumor and hoped they had eliminated the cancer completely from her body.

Shocking as the diagnosis was, it did not come as much of a surprise to Marlene or her doctors. Cysts and moles had been appearing on Marlene's body rather frequently over the previous ten years—a chalazion on her right eye, a lipoma on her back, a subcutaneous nodule on her back, a kerototic lesion on her chest, a pigmented lesion on her right palm. The list went on. These growths had been removed as they had appeared, and all had been benign. Nevertheless, each excision had been met with fearful anxiety.

Two years after her melanoma diagnosis, Marlene suffered acute abdominal pain that sent her to Massachusetts General Hospital in Boston. There, renowned Mass General surgeon Dr. A. Benedict Cosimi performed exploratory surgery and discovered that Marlene's small intestine had been "infiltrated extensively" by cancerous tumors. Dr. Cosimi removed twenty-two inches of her small intestine, excising as many tumors as possible. But the surgeon noted that the cancer had spread to other parts of her digestive tract and very likely to the lymph system and other organs. Little else could be done.

Metastatic melanoma is among the most lethal of all cancers and is considered incurable. The best Marlene could hope for was six months to a year of life. She and her husband, Keven, had four children.

Marlene's only medical option was to enroll in one of the experimental cancer treatments offered at several large cancer centers. As Dr. Cosimi noted in his report, it would be "reasonable for her to look into the interferon program at Yale."

Marlene did just that. She met with doctors and researchers at the Yale Medical Center in New Haven, Connecticut, and at the New England Medical Center and the Dana Farber Medical Center in Boston. Not only did the experimental treatments offer no evidence for a cure, but they gave little hope of extending her life. Furthermore, researchers from all three medical centers acknowledged that the side effects from the treatments would be significant, possibly even lethal.

After discussing the matter with Keven, Marlene declined the experimental treatments. She then gave up her job as associate vice president at a major stock brokerage firm in order to spend more time with her husband and four children, who ranged in age from nine to twenty.

In the weeks that followed, Marlene's condition quickly deteriorated. At five feet six inches tall, she weighed approximately ninety pounds. She was skin and bones. Her cheeks were dark hollows, her skin sallow and gray. Her eyes drooped with exhaustion. She was alive, but barely. Then something unexpected occurred. Marlene's brother, Albert, an engineer, showed up at Marlene's house, carrying grocery bags full of macrobiotic foods—a wide array of vegetables, brown rice, beans, and other staples— along with a book by Michio Kushi with Alex Jack entitled *The Cancer Prevention Diet*. Apparently, Albert had heard about the plant-based diet known as macrobiotics the day before, and had learned that people were using it to help them overcome a number of serious illnesses and conditions, including cancer.

"Albert, what is this stuff?" Marlene asked.

"These are macrobiotic foods," Albert said, unable to restrain his excitement. "Here," he said, handing her the book he had brought. "This book explains what it is all about."

Marlene looked at her brother incredulously. "Albert, I'm way beyond cancer prevention," she said. "I've moved on to cancer treatment."

"No, no," Albert said. "This book can help you now. It's about the cause of cancer and how you can use food to recover."

Marlene hadn't believed a word Albert had said, but his love and devotion had moved her.

"Okay," Marlene said. "I'll read the book tonight." She embraced her brother. "I love you. Thank you," she said.

The Cancer Prevention Diet made little impression on Marlene, and she had no interest in pursuing the diet. But Albert was already one step ahead of her. He had found a macrobiotic cook in Providence named Eileen Shea and insisted that Marlene speak to her. Again Marlene resisted, and again she surrendered to her brother's enthusiasm. At their initial meeting, Eileen referred Marlene to Dr. Marc Van Cauwenberghe, who counseled people in the macrobiotic approach to diet and health. One week later, at his office in Boston, Dr. Van Cauwenberghe examined Marlene and placed her on a strict macrobiotic diet that included vegetable soups, a wide variety of grains and beans, numerous daily servings of vegetables, a single daily serving of sea vegetables, and one serving of white fish each week.

Marlene was still not convinced of the possible efficacy of a dietary approach to cancer, but she had no other option left. She was dying, and Dr. Van Cauwenberghe seemed intelligent and sincere. He offered her hope. *What did she have to lose?* she asked herself.

Although she did not know it at the time, there was plenty of good scientific evidence to support the diet that she was about to adopt. Tens of thousands of substances in plant foods do, in fact, have powerful therapeutic value, especially in the fight against cancer and other major illnesses. But none of this information was part of Marlene's thinking at the moment of her decision. All she had to go on was an inner voice that told her to do it—and she did it with religious conviction. She followed Dr. Van Cauwenberghe's recommendations to the letter, and regularly consulted with him. Among the things Dr. Van Cauwenberghe told her was that her palate would change with time, and that she would begin truly enjoying the foods in her new diet. In fact, he suggested that the foods featured in her new diet would soon become the only kind she would crave.

To be sure, there were numerous factors present in Marlene's life that helped her sustain the diet and would later have a big impact on her health. The first, of course, was Eileen Shea, who prepared food for Marlene and gave her cooking classes. There was also a significant community of people that was using the macrobiotic diet to overcome their own serious illnesses. The social support Marlene received from those who were following the same diet was of incalculable value. So, too, was the fact that other members of the community had used the macrobiotic diet to overcome their own serious illnesses. It wasn't long before Marlene started to experience some small but significant changes.

Within weeks of adopting the diet, Marlene felt an unmistakable increase in energy. Her skin appeared to be getting brighter. She slept more deeply and restfully, and woke up with greater vitality. During the day, her mind was clearer and her memory better.

One change seemed particularly encouraging. Marlene had noticed that during the months preceding her diagnosis her menses were dark and thick. Two months after adopting the diet, she noticed that her menstrual blood had become bright red. Did these changes in color indicate that her blood now contained more oxygen and fewer toxins? The more Marlene thought about it, the more this conclusion made sense. More oxygen in the blood would explain the increase in energy, mental clarity, and improved skin tone. Could other benefits be possible? Could blood that is richer in oxygen and less burdened by impurities be better for her immune system?

Marlene began taking short walks every day. She attended a gym twice a week and, with the help of a trainer, worked out with a five-pound bar, which was all she could lift. She did some gentle exercises on the resistance equipment and received a light massage from a shiatsu therapist once a week. She also got lots of help in her daily life. A retired emergency room nurse helped her with her housekeeping and shopping; friends ran errands for her; and others picked up her children when she was tired or had to visit her doctor.

Marlene also made a deeper connection to her religious roots in Roman Catholicism. She prayed daily, attended church, and regularly visited La Salette, a shrine devoted to the Virgin Mary, located in Attleboro, Massachusetts, just thirty minutes from her home. As her spirituality deepened, Marlene began to see her diet and other healing behaviors as a form of spiritual practice. She was fasting without the pain of hunger; she was exercising to cleanse her body of impurities; she was slowing down and bringing her awareness to her inner life; she was spending time with her husband and children because love was what mattered most to her now.

Meanwhile, she had monthly blood tests taken to monitor her condition. Her doctors expected the tests to reveal that her cancer was advancing. But after three months on the macrobiotic diet, Marlene's blood tests had all returned to normal, including those for cancer. After six months on the diet, there was no denying that she was getting better. She was no longer losing weight. She was experiencing remarkable energy. Her stamina and strength were growing. Her blood tests remained normal and, in some cases, even became ideal. In fact, according to her blood work, there seemed to be no sign of cancer anywhere in her body.

Marlene wanted to know definitively whether or not she still had cancer. She asked her doctor to tell her which test would give the most accurate diagnosis? An MRI, her doctor said. An MRI, or magnetic resonance imaging test, uses a magnetic field and radio waves to create precise pictures of organs and structures within the body. The test can detect abnormalities in the body that cannot be seen on x-rays, ultrasounds, or computer tomography (CT) scans. An MRI, her doctor said, could detect the presence of tumors in her body.

"Please schedule that test," Marlene asked.

The physician urged caution. No doubt, there were still tumors in her intestinal tract that Dr. Cosimi had not removed, and very likely there would be others, located elsewhere in her body, in her lymph system and perhaps in her liver. "Was she sure she wanted such information?" her doctor asked. Marlene thought about it for a moment and then said, "Yes."

The MRI was done at Massachusetts General Hospital seven months after Marlene had begun following the macrobiotic diet under Marc Van Cauwenberghe's guidance. The test results were unequivocal. There were no signs of cancer anywhere in her body. Marlene went on to write a book, *When Hope Never Dies*, about her experience of overcoming malignant melanoma. She has since given countless lectures, spoken at dozens of conferences, and personally guided many people back to health.

OVERCOMING YOUR FEAR

To be shocked is to be overwhelmed with fear. Those who have been diagnosed with a life-threatening illness say that their fear, at least initially, seemed limitless, like falling into a darkened chasm that had no bottom. For most, such a diagnosis is followed by a period of grim detachment.

Many become numb, others overcome by despair. All previous interests and preoccupations seem to have little to no importance. Former duties that once seemed essential soon feel grotesquely irrelevant.

No one can rationally deal with a diagnosis of a terminal disease. Shock is a kind of protective reaction, a form of cocooning, in the face of the overwhelming nature of the events and the feelings exploding inside. Shock dims the conscious mind while allowing the unconscious processes to do their job, which is to rearrange your inner life on the basis of this new information. A new identity is being forged, one that can better cope with the current realities. The numbness that characterizes this period is a kind of anesthetic, allowing profound changes to occur inside of you, even without your being aware.

The question is this: What do you do while you are still in shock? Some of those who beat the odds say that the best thing to do is to rest and let others care for you as best they can. Meanwhile, stay open to the unexpected occurrences that may offer glimmers of hope. Life is full of mystery. No one can predict the future. A doctor may know the odds of recovery based on population studies, but your future is a complete mystery, the details of which are absolutely unknown. Hold on to that fact. As you will see, there will be lots of positive actions that you can take when the time is right. But at this first stage, this state of shock, fighting the good fight means engaging in small acts of self-care, resting, and allowing others to help you. As tiny as these measures may seem, they are, in fact, acts of defiance against surrender.

Surrender can lead to depression, which, in turn, can weaken your immune system. A study published in the British medical journal *The Lancet* demonstrated that prolonged depression was associated with significantly decreased immune response, including weakened natural killer cells, which target and destroy cancer cells. Similarly, researchers have known for decades that bereavement—a natural and healthy response to the loss of a loved one—can, if not coped with in a healthy way, lead to depression, which in turn can weaken the immune system and increase susceptibility to disease and even death. Those who suffer from prolonged bereavement with accompanying depression experience far higher rates of mortality in their respective age groups than those who have not experienced such a loss.

In a Mount Sinai Hospital study, Dr. Steven Schleifer and his colleagues discovered that bereavement caused a deadening effect on a specific type of immune cell, called a lymphocyte, which failed to react in the presence of a pathogen or aberrant cell. Other studies at Mount Sinai have suggested that bereavement also impairs the hypothalamus, an area in the brain that has an enormous influence on the endocrine and immune systems. Schleifer concluded that, in the face of such loss, many people give up the will to live. The body's defenses weaken, increasing the likelihood of premature death.

In time, however, the immune system can right itself, especially when people get the help they need to heal emotionally. With the right support, the immune system can reemerge from its weakened state and oftentimes restore itself to normal function, which demonstrates how important it is to maintain hope, especially during the first few months after disease has been discovered. In time, your inner life can grow stronger and better able to deal with the trauma of the diagnosis. Little by little, shock gives way to emerging rays of clarity. A new state of balance is achieved, one that is more accepting and free of excessive fear.

Virtually everyone I have spoken to who has been diagnosed with a terrible illness eventually arrives at this inner state of equilibrium. What people often do not realize is that the changes that have occurred unconsciously have brought about an entirely new vision of life that is itself more balanced and humble. Many people appreciate their loved ones as never before. They awaken to small expressions of love and feel a new sense of gratitude. Often they seek out the beauty and nourishing richness of nature, and find themselves marveling at seemingly ordinary events—a bird in flight, the morning sun, or a soft breeze. Despite all the pain they are going through, they see life through new eyes and with a new perspective.

A Belgian man who overcame prostate cancer by using a plant-based diet and other natural methods once told me that his illness set him on a journey that enriched every aspect of his life. "At first, I was shocked and terrified, of course," he said. "But as I learned more and applied all kinds of new forms of knowledge, my whole life improved. In time, I realized that the tumor was my friend. It had led me to a better life."

A confrontation with death alters a person's life and character, a transformation that makes the first step in the healing journey possible. The central character change that takes place at this step is a transition from shock to a humble, loving, and compassionate relationship with yourself and those around you. This step requires you to slow down, bring your gentle awareness back to yourself, and reestablish intimacy with your inner life. This change becomes the foundation for the entire healing journey.

COMPASSION VS. SELF-PITY

Compassion is not self-pity, though people often confuse the two. Self-pity is laced with feelings of powerlessness, self-criticism, anger at oneself and others, and even self-hatred. As a powerless victim, one is unable to take any kind of positive, corrective action. Compassion, on the other hand, is infused with gentle love for oneself and others. One becomes aware of the universal nature of suffering and our shared vulnerability. There is nobility and honesty in compassion. And perhaps most telling of all, there is the power to take remedial action. In the end, the compassionate heart is a warrior's heart that seeks to make the world a better place for oneself and others.

With compassion comes humility, which frees us from the burden of pride. That alone makes us more open, freer of bias, and more capable of receiving new information. In our humility, we are also grateful and open-hearted. We can be inspired by others and by new ideas.

In fact, humility and compassion are the natural responses to illness or injury. Even the common cold has the capacity to humble us, to put us flat on our backs, to make us forget the outside world and instead turn our attention and care to ourselves. Turning inward with care and love is the natural response to illness. When your body is wounded or hurting, you need care, and that care must come with love.

Creating a compassionate relationship with one's self is not always easy, though. Indeed, many of us believe that the ideal behavior at this time is to deny the pain of diagnosis, to march stoically on, and to ask for as little as possible—in short, to become invisible. Others take a different approach. Their anger and regret are expressed outwardly as bitter complaining that alienates everyone around them. The results of such complaining are so predictable that we can only wonder if those who indulge in the practice secretly seek the very rejection they inevitably receive. It is as if they are asking others to confirm their own belief that they are unworthy of love.

Feelings of unworthiness, self-criticism, and the harmful behaviors that inevitably come with such feelings only cause more hurt. This is not the time for more pain. The healing forces within you must be supported. And the state of mind and heart that does this best is compassion.

But how does one learn compassion, especially in a hurry? Perhaps the answer is that you don't have to learn compassion at all. Maybe it's something you already know.

FINDING COMPASSION AND HEALING LOVE

Living deep within the human psyche are powerful spiritual energies and sources of instinct, knowledge, and wisdom that we all share as part of our human inheritance. Included in this collection of instinctual states are our innate need for love, our biological preference for beauty, our fear of the dark, and the wonder and balance we experience when in nature. Among the most powerful of these sources of wisdom and healing is the archetypal mother.

The archetypal mother is the source of maternal instincts. It gives women an innate wisdom that guides them through motherhood, especially during pregnancy and the early years of a child's life. It also exists in men, especially in stay-at-home fathers who serve as primary caregivers of infants. In both women and men, the archetypal mother informs the ability to nurture and heal. This archetype also serves as a guiding light that shows us where to turn when we are hurt or ill. Indeed, every child knows to run to his or her mother—the earthly manifestation of the archetype—whenever he or she is ill or has been injured.

Even modern medicine, with its overwhelming emphasis on the intellectual, has been unable to repress this basic, instinctual need for this wise, heart-centered healing force. When you are afraid and in need of healing, you yearn for the comfort, care, patience, and wisdom that flow from the archetypal mother.

The archetypal mother is a fundamental, ancient image, containing within itself vast wisdom and instinctual knowledge. This image lives in the unconscious and is manifest in stories, myths, and fairy tales. People draw from this ancient well to varying degrees, which is why we all seem to differ so dramatically in our abilities to serve as mothers, nurturers, or healers.

Traditionally, archetypes were often worshipped as deities, and the archetypal mother was no exception. Throughout human history, she has been referred to as the Divine Mother, the Goddess, the Divine Feminine, and the Holy Mother. She was embodied by various figures in many of the world's religions—Mary in the New Testament, Kuan Yin in Buddhism, Parvati in Hinduism, Sophia in the Old Testament, and Hera (and many others) in Greek mythology. In religious contexts, the Divine Mother is the source of all regeneration. It is the mother who, after the barrenness of winter, gives birth to the renewal of spring. Her love is the power behind all forms of restoration, fertility, healing, and rebirth. She has the power to give life.

Your biological mother is an earthly manifestation of the Divine Mother, who, to whatever degree she was capable, channeled the love and wisdom of the archetype. Your biological mother gave you life. She is the source of your physical existence. Indeed, you grew a body and received your earliest psychological training inside her womb, where her blood was your blood, and where you shared many of her emotional and psychological states. When you were born, your fundamental needs for food, water, warmth, cleanliness, and understanding rested to a great extent on your mother's love, wisdom, and actions. Did your mother respond with love when, for example, you needed holding, or rest, or food, or sleep, or warmth, or bathing, or a change of diaper? Or was she distracted or overcome by her own internal conflicts? Your experience in these formative years determined, to a great extent, how you feel about your needs, and whether you believe you deserve to be cared for or are worthy of love.

The challenge most of us face is that we were given mixed messages from our mothers and fathers regarding how we should feel about our own physical and emotional needs. Examples of this conflicted state abound. Mothers who are ill, or depressed, or psychologically challenged very often experience enormous ambivalence whenever their children need care. They don't have the capacity to focus their love and attention on their children's needs because they are overwhelmed by their own. Under the stress of desperate emotions, young mothers can pull away from their children or act out emotionally, especially when the children's needs become demanding.

The psychological scarring for both child and parent is terrible. Many children grow up feeling that their needs were the cause of their mothers' pain, stress, and unhappiness. Some children respond to these beliefs by denying their own needs, wishing that they were invisible or didn't exist at all.

If have recently discovered you are seriously ill, this is not the time to deny the need for care, understanding, and love—all of which must take precedence over any negative training you may have received during childhood or maintained as an adult. This is the moment to open your heart, grow in compassion for yourself and others, and adopt new behaviors that can help you heal. Among the first and most practical ways of overcoming negative childhood training is to experience regularly the Divine Mother, who is a source of compassion, healing, and unconditional love. There is neither criticism nor blame from the Divine Mother. There is only love and understanding—an understanding that transcends your own. When you might criticize yourself, she will not. Even the mistakes you feel are obvious and perhaps warrant some form of retribution, she refuses to condemn. She is unconditional love personified.

What does such love and compassion look like? How can it be channeled into your daily life now? One of its clearest expressions in modern times was Mother Teresa of Calcutta, who in 2016 was named a saint by the Roman Catholic Church. She said the following in her acceptance speech for the 1979 Nobel Peace Prize:

"One evening we went out and we picked up four people from the street," Mother Teresa said. "And one of them was in a most terrible condition. And I told the sisters, 'You take care of the other three; I will take care of this one that looks worse.' So I did for her all that my love can do. I put her in bed, and there was such a beautiful smile on her face. She took hold of my hand, as she said one word only—'Thank you'—and she died.

"I could not help but examine my conscience before her. And I asked, 'What would I say if I was in her place?' And my answer was very simple. I would have tried to draw a little attention to myself. I would have said, 'I am hungry, I am dying, I am cold, I am in pain,' or something. But she gave me much more—she gave me her grateful love. And she died with a smile on her face, like that man who we picked up from the drain, half eaten with worms, and we brought him to the home—'I have lived like an animal in the street,' [he said] 'but I am going to die like an angel, loved and cared for.' And it was so wonderful to see the greatness of that man who could speak like that, who could die like that without blaming, without cursing anybody, without comparing anything—like an angel. This is the greatness of our people."

Mother Teresa did not ask this woman or that man how they came to be in such straits. She did not blame them for their suffering, nor wonder what they might have done to experience such harrowing circumstances. She did not ask about their backgrounds. Such thoughts arise from the intellectual center, and thus are entirely foreign to the heart-centered consciousness. Acting from the heart, Mother Teresa identified with the suffering ("What would I do if I were in her place?") and gave each of them exactly what they needed in the moment: unconditional love in the form of a bath, rest, food, and loving care. She embodied compassion. Indeed, she was the living version of the archetypal mother.

The Divine Mother helps us make the shift from intellectually centered to heart-centered consciousness—from criticism to compassion. The mother, present within each of us, facilitates this shift by showing us a way of being that is beyond criticism, judgment, fear, and feelings of unworthiness.

We can call upon the Divine Mother by asking in prayer or meditation for help and healing. One way to feel this presence is to ask yourself how the Divine Mother would treat you if you were in pain? If you need a real-life example, ask yourself this question: How would Mother Teresa treat me now? By asking the question honestly and sincerely, you will experience a shift in your awareness. You will feel the love of the Divine Mother that is within you. This love can cause you to relax and settle more fully into your body, into the wisdom of your heart, and into the present moment. You can practically feel a spiritual presence embracing you, awakening you to the love that flows within you. This compassionate aspect of your being can permeate your life and guide your actions, especially when you need rest, or while you care for your body, or speak to someone you love.

The archetypal mother's powers flow naturally into strong healers, both men and women. Indeed, the mother's healing abilities are what imbue the true nurse, who combines compassion, a healing touch, courage, and medical expertise. When combined in a single person, these characteristics represent a rare degree of psychological integration. Such a person is able to hold within the loftiest characteristics of humanity as well as a practical knowledge of what to do in a crisis. Like the mother, the true healer is free of any trace of inner critic. She does not blame you for your illness or injury. Her consciousness is rooted in the absolute now. Her only interest is in your immediate needs, and in how your suffering and illness can be overcome.

As much as possible, do for yourself what that true healer would do for you. In addition, ask others to do what they can to help you now. If you continue to act as a good healer toward yourself—that is to say, to act non-judgmentally and non-critically—you will recognize a good healer when one shows up in your life.

THE PRESENT MOMENT

Many people who have overcome serious illnesses have told me that they had lost track of themselves prior to becoming sick. They had allowed the daily demands and their hectic schedules to steal their lives, drastically increasing their stress levels and making it difficult, if not impossible, to stay aware of their own needs and limitations. When we are too absorbed in the moment-to-moment pressures of our daily affairs, we very rarely, if ever, take time to wonder, *What do I need now? How do I feel? What is my body asking me for?*

The harried nature of such an existence prevents us from knowing our needs and the needs of those we love. The most important parts of our lives go unnourished. This loss of self elevates stress levels, allows symptoms to go unheeded, and eventually contributes to the onset of disease, according to those who have restored themselves to health. As one person put it, "You can't neglect yourself and all that you are suffering without eventually causing some kind of breakdown."

The compassion and unconditional love of the archetypal mother brings you back to intimacy with yourself and to what is essential in life. Coming back to yourself and the immediate present is an act of healing and self-love. It makes you more attuned to yourself, your environment, and the lives of those you love. In Buddhism, the practice is referred to as mindfulness. It is being aware of yourself, your feelings, your body in the here-and-now, without reacting to those feelings with any judgment.

As you come back to the present, you may experience a deeper state of relaxation. Your breathing and heart rate very likely will slow down. Subtle changes in your biology may occur. Your body will relax; your muscles will release some of their tension. Your blood will better circulate oxygen and release carbon dioxide. As you learn to relax even more, you will experience a deepening connection with your inner life. Your mood will elevate. Your heart will open. You may become aware of certain intangible aspects of your being, parts of you that can be described only as spirit or soul. These are just some of the benefits of communing with your inner life, and especially with the archetypal or Divine Mother within you.

The Divine Mother teaches you to listen without having to change anything. You are encouraged merely to be aware of what you feel and to hold those feelings with compassion.

To do this, you need time every day to sit with your thoughts and feelings and allow them to exist without censorship or criticism. Soon this powerful healing tool—simply being with your feelings without judgment or the need to change them—will turn into practical, daily behaviors that follow from a spirit of compassion and love.

WHAT TO DO NOW

There are a number of small healing acts that can bring the archetypal mother's healing love and wisdom into your life on a daily basis. Adopt these habits and you will find yourself taking the first step of your journey of healing successfully.

Create Gaps in Time

Take some time every day to sit comfortably and allow yourself to witness your thoughts and whatever you are feeling physically and emotionally. Bring your loving, compassionate awareness to your physical sensations, emotions, and thoughts. Do not judge your sensations, thoughts, or feelings. Do not let your intellect assess or label your current state. Indeed, whatever you are feeling will change in time, and the fact is that you do not know how things will change. Allow yourself not to know. Simply remain open. Observe your thoughts and experience what you feel physically and emotionally. Hold these thoughts and sensations with the mother's kindness, compassion, and non-judgment. As you observe your feelings with compassion, let each sensation, thought, and emotion pass through your awareness. Breathe and let go. When you find yourself engaging an emotion, especially fear or anger, try to bring your awareness back to your breath.

This act requires nothing more than to sit comfortably in the sun and be aware of what you are feeling. As fear, anger, or sadness arises, you can gently breathe soothing love into those emotions, and into the places in the body where those feelings are held. There is no work involved. You are simply allowing your own existence to become the object of your awareness. As your life emerges into your consciousness and you become aware of the Divine Mother's love, something odd and wonderful can happen. You may experience yourself relaxing deeply and being held in a feeling of soft grace, as if a larger force within you were opening its wings and surrounding you with peace and harmony.

In these moments, you will likely receive new insights into your life, activities, and relationships. Note these revelations. Remember them, but put them on the shelf for later consideration. Many of them may be important. Follow up later. In these moments, peace and tranquility are your only goals. Release every negative thought. Be restored to the present moment. Come back to your breath, to the rise and fall of your chest, to the feeling of relaxation, to the enjoyment of the here and now.

Act with Compassion

In your old life, before your diagnosis, many of your activities may have been done with the intention of completing each job so that you could move on to the next thing on your "to-do" list—whether it was your next project or assignment, or the next item on your grocery list. Your mind may have been focused on getting to the end of the list rather than on the individual actions themselves. This mindset must be changed.

It's time to slow down and gently focus your awareness on whatever you are doing in the here and now. As you engage in an activity, try to imbue any action you take with as much kindness, compassion, and love as you can. Become more deeply aware of what you are doing and the attitude with which you are doing it. Focus on the action rather than the results of the action. To do so, you will have to slow down a little and release yourself from timelines, deadlines, and any pressure to excel.

Even the simplest act can be done with gentle, soothing awareness. Your every act must be done with a certain kindness that flows from your heart-centered awareness and into the action itself. Doing your job, cleaning your house, doing the laundry, cooking and eating your food, choosing the kind of music you listen to, interacting with those you love—everything can be done slowly, consciously, and in a healing way. Throughout your day, notice how this awareness affects what you do, your every thought and emotion, and your every interaction with others. This awareness will help you choose more carefully the kinds of events you participate in, and the people with whom you spend time. Eliminate events that drain you. Avoid people who take too much of your energy or good will, or who engage in negative thinking that may weaken your life condition.

Self-knowledge and the need to treat yourself with kindness and compassion must now become the basis for your every choice in life. Do your best to make wise choices.

Walk in Nature

Every time we walk in a forest or by the ocean, or sit by a river or lake, we are communing with the Divine Mother. Nature, the living expression of the Divine Mother, overwhelms us with its gentle, healing energy. As so many of us have experienced, it's nearly impossible to sit by a river or walk by the ocean and maintain negative or critical thoughts. Eventually, nature overpowers our fears and anger and replaces them with a sense of balance, stillness, and peace.

If you can't get to a park or some other natural environment, take short, gentle walks in your neighborhood. Don't power walk and don't exhaust yourself. Rather, walk with an awareness of your body's needs and feelings. Gently establish a rhythm that is in harmony with the level of energy you are experiencing at that particular moment. As your energy rises, you will increase the pace; as it wanes, you'll slow down and stroll. Stay connected to yourself and walk in harmony with your energy levels and your inner life.

Walking is the ideal exercise. You may begin walking while feeling burdened by your cares and concerns, but as you continue, you will very likely feel relieved of the intensity of these concerns. By the time you get home, you may experience a great deal of relief, clarity, and equilibrium.

Write from the Heart

Writing in a diary can be a healing exercise, especially if you write in your compassionate voice. As you write, try to become intimate with your own suffering—that is to say, turn your awareness to your symptoms, fears, anger, or conflicts while at the same time holding feelings of care and love for yourself. Write with a compassionate heart, experiencing your suffering without judging yourself. Tap into the archetypal mother's love. Your intention should simply be to become aware of your anger, sadness, and fear. Allow these feelings to emerge and hold them with compassion and understanding. You will feel any negative judgments pass like dark clouds being swept away by the wind. You will be left feeling deeply relieved, clear, and free of inner conflict.

As much as you can, try to find reasons for gratitude in whatever you are writing about, especially in the small or large victories you may experience. Acknowledge each positive experience as a blessing on the healing path. Gratitude can have the mysterious effect of multiplying the blessings and the victories. It will also enhance your ability to see even more reasons for gratitude. As your gratitude for small blessings grows, you may also recognize these positive events as subtle evidence of an unseen force that is assisting you in your efforts to heal. Acknowledgment of this force can strengthen your faith, and as we will see later in this book, your faith can, in turn, strengthen your immune system and healing forces.

See a Healer

At this stage in the healing process, you may wish to see a practitioner of some form of complementary medicine, a person who can provide gentle healing touch and support without asking you to alter your current behavior. It's more important to be understood and supported than to be criticized and encouraged to change. Seek out a healer who is understanding, compassionate, and loving—one who is capable of channeling that love through touch alone. There are many forms of gentle healing touch, including Reiki, acupressure, therapeutic massage, and Jin Shin Jyutsu. Each one can be extremely healing, but in the end, the compassion, depth of understanding, and experience of the practitioner is more important than the specific practice.

Teachers and other healers will show up later on your path of healing when you are prepared to take up new healing tools and change old patterns. But at this moment, you may feel a need to rest in someone's compassionate understanding. Healing touch and compassionate listening is more important to you than advice.

Engage in Conscious Movement

The mother's awareness and compassion can be brought to the body through the practice of stretching, dance, yoga, or gentle martial arts—specifically, the ancient Chinese practices of qi gong or tai chi chuan. Whether you stretch, or dance, or learn tai chi, the awareness with which you do the exercise is the same: Connect in kindness with your body. Your intention is not to achieve the perfect posture, but rather to embrace your body with intimacy, care, and love. Many YMCAs and community centers offer different forms of healing movement classes, including dance, yoga, tai chi, and qi gong.

Walking slowly, consciously, and mindfully can become a meditation on your love and compassion for your body and entire being, as you experience your strengths and accept and appreciate your limits.

Pray and Meditate

By directing your prayers toward the Divine Mother, or by using guided imagery and meditation to become aware of your feelings, you can bring great peace and balance to your inner life. Mindfulness can help us deal very effectively with fear and anger, the two big emotions that, if allowed to, could drive any of us mad at this point. One of the best ways to deal with these negative emotions is to do the following meditation, which can lead you from fear and anger to sadness, compassion, and self-love.

Begin by sitting comfortably in a quiet room in your home. If possible, light a candle, or two candles, to create a feeling of intimacy and calm. Close your eyes and relax. Breathe from your belly, inhaling through your nose with your mouth closed, allowing the air to fill your chest. Exhale through your nose. With each outward breath, envision yourself releasing as much tension as you can from your body. Feel your body relax. As you become more aware of your body, your mind and body will relax together and become more intimately linked. Each will support the other in the relaxation process. Once you feel deeply relaxed, you may then proceed to the next step.

Without creating any image or attaching yourself to any that might emerge, embrace your fear. Be aware of the fear, as if you were looking at it without judging it, without repressing it. At first, you will notice that your fear will increase. Stay with it. Keep breathing from your belly, inhaling and exhaling deeply. Your awareness—meaning your pure conscious attention without judgment—has the power to dissolve your fear. Witness your fear without attaching to it, as if it were a passing cloud. You are bigger than your fear. Your life is of greater importance than anyone has taught you to believe. You are more than the image or identity you have made of yourself.

As you continue to meditate on your inner state, you will likely become aware that your fear is retreating. As it does, you may find that your fear is now replaced by anger. Continue to breathe deeply, emphasizing your exhalations as you release your tension. Allow the anger to rise within you. Feel it. Allow yourself to express your anger if you feel the need to do so. Punch a pillow. Yell into a pillow. Pray. Direct your anger toward its source—even at God, if that's who is making you angry. Stay with your anger, keeping your eyes closed and breathing deeply. Hold your anger in your awareness just as you did with your fear, without guilt or judgment, without getting attached for very long to any image that may arise in your mind.

At some point, you will start to feel trapped by your anger as it reaches a peak. You will recognize that all your decisions have led you to this point in your life. There was no escaping this moment. Each one of your choices cascaded into the next, which fell into the next, so that it felt as if there were never any choices at all, but just an endless string of events that led you to this time.

You are not to blame for being in these circumstances. Life brought you to this moment and there was no escaping it. When you allow yourself to feel and perhaps express your anger, you will feel trapped. When this feeling of being trapped reaches its peak, it will naturally change into sadness— a pure and cleansing sadness that, for many, will translate into tears. Allow your tears to flow. Crying is one of the body's ways of releasing stagnant emotions and rearranging long-standing, blocked energy patterns. As you cry, your sadness will quickly fall into deeper feelings of compassion for yourself. Continue to breathe. At this point, you will be awakening to your tenderness, your vulnerability, and your courage. You have done the best you could with your life. Embrace yourself with that compassion and care. Go deeply into that compassion and know that you are being held, without any judgment, by the living energies that are, at this very moment, communicating love to you. Allow yourself to tumble into this love. Feel the depth of it. Feel its unconditional nature. Know that this great love embraces you, infusing you with compassion and the experience of being cared for and understood. This love and compassion are, in fact, powerful healing energies. They are also the basis for hope.

Don't be alarmed or critical of yourself if you do not pass through every level of this meditation. Continue to practice it without judgment or any trace of self-criticism. The key to this meditation is to get to your sadness, allow yourself to release your pain as tears, and fall into that inner state of compassion for yourself.

THE POWER OF SMALL BLESSINGS

Positive actions, however small they may be, and the positive feelings they evoke, can have a powerful effect on your immune and healing forces. According to research conducted by Dr. Arthur Stone, a psychologist at the medical school of the State University of New York at Stony Brook, a single pleasurable event can boost the immune system for as much as two days. Conversely, negative events, such as criticism, especially from a superior or one's employer, can depress immune function for up to twenty-four hours, thus making people more vulnerable to illness.

"Positive events of the day seem to have a stronger helpful impact on immune function than upsetting events do a negative one," Dr. Stone told the *New York Times*. "Having a good time on Monday still had a positive effect on the immune system by Wednesday," Dr. Stone said. "But the negative immune effect from undesirable events on Monday lasts just for that day."

The most powerful effects on immune response, Dr. Stone found, resulted from positive solitary activities, such as fishing or jogging. On the other hand, when study participants were criticized by an employer, suffered a difficult encounter with a coworker, or experienced prolonged stress at work, they experienced a diminution of their immune response for the duration of the next day.

You may be tempted to fall into negative emotions and neglect your need for small pleasures throughout your day. Don't succumb to such temptations. Do whatever you can to experience fun and enjoyment—see a good film, laugh whenever possible, enjoy a good talk with someone you love, take a walk, or commune with the world of spirit. These small acts of self-nurturance and compassion can bring you to a new state of emotional stability. Indeed, they can get you past the shock and help you develop a new healing relationship with yourself. They can also have very real effects on your healing forces.

In a short while, you will start to feel stronger, at which point you will want to do more for your healing. As this desire increases, doors will start to open in your mind and heart. You will realize that there is a lot you can do to help yourself and promote your healing. That's when you will know that you are ready for the second step on your healing journey.

*T*AKE BACK YOUR POWER

Little steps soon lead to bigger ones. Like tiny seeds planted in the soil of your consciousness, small acts of compassion directed toward yourself and others can begin to change the way you think, feel, and behave. Miraculously, this very compassion can bring greater emotional and psychological stability to you. Before long you may realize that you are getting emotionally stronger, perhaps a little more focused, a little more determined. You may feel ready to participate more fully in your healing process. That's when the necessity for step two will dawn on you—the moment you realize you must be directly involved in every decision that relates to your healing. You must take back your power and become truly responsible for your recovery.

At the beginning of step two, information is of paramount importance. You must learn as much as you can about your illness. Books, articles, relevant websites on the internet, and the National Institutes of Health Medical online library, known as PubMed, are all good sources of information. (See Resources on page 217.) The experiences of others who have faced the same disease as your own or similar illnesses are also important. You should vary your sources as much as possible simply because you must distinguish between relevant information and material that has no value.

Listen to your doctor's treatment plan and medical advice, and ask as many questions as are necessary. At the same time, you must widen your search for answers beyond the standard medical approach to include complementary healing modalities that have the potential to improve your chances of recovery and enhance the quality of your life.

You will want to know how you can determine if any single medical or complementary approach is working. It's important to be able to assess the efficacy of both orthodox and complementary methods. If something isn't working, you will want to stop using it. If it is working, you'll want to take full advantage of it by utilizing it with as much consistency and enthusiasm as possible.

You can gauge your program in several ways. The first is through medical tests, including blood and urine analyses, which you will do with your doctor. Another way is to consult your doctor regularly on his or her assessment of your condition and progress. The same can be done with your complementary healers. You should also ask yourself how you feel on a daily basis, and how each treatment may be affecting you. Some people like to keep a healing journal in which they record their feelings, any changes in their condition, and self-assessments on a regular basis. As your treatment plan broadens to include more complementary therapies, you will want to keep track of how each approach affects you physically, emotionally, and mentally.

In the chapters that follow, you will find a wide array of effective complementary approaches that can form the foundation of your complementary program, as well as scientific and medical research that supports the use of each modality. You will find that the experiences of people who have used these approaches often reveal how effective the combination of medical and complementary healing programs can be. The more engaged you become in the search for answers, the more you will find yourself gaining in personal power and confidence. The deeper rewards of this step will open up to you. As your confidence grows, you will be able to infuse your every treatment with a deeper, richer, and more healing faith. You will stop being a passive recipient of medical treatment and instead become an engaged, active, co-healer in your own recovery process.

Those who get well look back on this step as a pivotal moment in their healing journeys. They realize that this step opened their minds and hearts to many important healing methods that later proved essential. Opening your heart and your mind awakens you to other dimensions of life. As you engage yourself more deeply in the healing process, you feel guided by gentle intimations and larger forces that are leading the way. But at this stage in the process you must be the one who takes the initiative and assumes responsibility for the work only you can do.

I can think of no better example of this step than Nathan Pritikin, the quintessential self-healing pioneer.

NATHAN PRITIKIN: TRAILBLAZER

Nathan Pritikin was a brilliant scientist and inventor who held more than sixty patents in electronics, chemistry, and engineering. Not only did he invent new technologies, but he also manufactured his inventions, which made him a very successful man. Pritikin had attended only two years of college at the University of Chicago, but used to say that he was better off for not having had a formal education. "If I had had more education, I'd be trapped into thinking like everyone else thought," he said. "Without so much training, I could explore scientific questions with a fresh view of things." This approach to problem solving served him well in life, especially after he was diagnosed with life-threatening heart disease.

The healing program that Nathan Pritikin would eventually create— one that would restore health to hundreds of thousands of patients with heart disease and other major illnesses—is today known to be safe and effective. But in the middle of the twentieth century, Pritikin's ideas seemed dangerous to medical doctors, even though the scientific evidence at the time supported his approach. In this way, Pritikin's story illustrates how scientific knowledge takes time to trickle down to medical practitioners, and how certain ideas can seem foreign or frightening to one generation but sensible and even obvious to the next.

On February 11, 1958, Pritikin, who was forty-three years old at the time, underwent testing at the Sansum Medical Clinic in Santa Barbara, California, and was diagnosed with coronary heart disease, meaning that cholesterol plaques, or atherosclerosis, had infiltrated the arteries leading to his heart, and that his heart had begun to suffocate for lack of oxygen. Atherosclerosis is the primary cause of most heart attacks and strokes. Pritikin's doctor prescribed atropine, a drug that increases heart rate and blood flow by stimulating the vagus nerve in the chest and neck. Pritikin was also ordered to limit his walking to the equivalent of four blocks per day, to take a nap every afternoon, and to eliminate all strenuous activity, including bicycle riding and tennis, two activities he had come to enjoy. His doctor told him that he should consider retiring from his business because it was far too stressful on his heart.

"Is this the only treatment?" Pritikin asked. "Don't you want me to change my diet or do something else to cure the illness?"

"No," his doctor told him. "Heart disease is incurable."

"What do you believe is the cause?" Pritikin wanted to know.

"Heart disease, cancer, and other degenerative illnesses are the natural consequences of aging and stress," his doctor informed him. "There's nothing that anyone can do to avoid them."

Nathan could not believe his ears. The doctor warned him that if he did not follow the recommendations, he would be risking a fatal heart attack.

Pritikin quickly abandoned the atropine after he found that the drug caused his eyes to dilate and forced him to wear sunglasses. Walking any distance terrified him and he curtailed all physical activity. As for the naps, occasionally he forced himself to take one.

Pritikin was no ordinary heart patient, though. He had been studying the relationship between diet and health—especially diet's connection to heart disease—since the late 1940s, when he discovered a little known series of potentially life-changing studies. According to the research, Europeans who had been placed on food rationing by the Nazis during World War II experienced a dramatic decline in heart disease deaths. Ironically, the food rationing arose because German soldiers had taken the meat, eggs, cheese and milk for themselves, and had forced the occupied people to eat a traditional peasant diet of barley, bread, potatoes, garden vegetables, and fruit.

After the war ended, European scientists discovered that during the war years, and for some time afterward, countries whose populations had been on this peasant diet had experienced very low rates of heart disease, despite the fact that these people had lived under tremendous stress. Autopsy studies done just after the war showed a remarkable absence of atherosclerosis in the coronary arteries of the occupied people.

Pritikin was among the small minority of scientists who saw the connection between the rationed diet and the healthy hearts. After further study, he learned that people around the world who ate their own version of the peasant diet—one composed mostly of vegetables, cooked whole grains, and fruit—also had low rates of heart disease, cancer, diabetes, and other serious illnesses. Animal studies revealed that blood cholesterol might be the key. High cholesterol was associated with heart disease, while low cholesterol was associated with good health. Pritikin theorized that by lowering his cholesterol levels, he might be able to cure himself of heart disease.

At the time, Pritikin ate as every other American did. He was particularly fond of ice cream, of which he ate a pint every night. But when he was diagnosed with heart disease and told to retire, he changed his eating habits. Guided by the research on occupied Europeans, Pritikin adopted his own version of the peasant diet, eating an abundance of green and leafy vegetables, root and sweet vegetables, beans, whole grains, and fruit.

He eliminated all red meat, dairy products, eggs, and chicken. For protein, he ate beans and small amounts of fish.

Pritikin's doctor was alarmed by his dietary changes. He told his patient that if he continued on this regimen, he would deprive his body of essential nutrients and would soon become sick. Pritikin decided to consult a nutritionist at the University of California, Los Angeles (UCLA). He described his diet and his plan to treat his heart disease by lowering his cholesterol level. The nutritionist was appalled. Foods high in fat and cholesterol are "the best foods you can eat," the nutritionist said. "We can't help you. It's too dangerous. You might kill yourself." Undeterred, Pritikin responded by becoming even more daring with his regimen. He engaged in lengthy experiments to see how individual foods affected his blood cholesterol level.

Meanwhile, he kept meticulous records. "Eating 10 dates after dinner," he wrote as one of his entries. "Start fruit at 1,000 calories 55 percent total intake," he wrote in another. On another occasion, he noted, "Three weeks on fruit at 55 to 60 percent of total calories, 1,000–1,200 calories fruit." Every telltale reaction he experienced was recorded: "22 days on dried fruit, 12 dates, 60 percent calories on dried fruit; calories 1,800, was thirsty last two weeks, constant dry taste in mouth." For a week, he ate nothing but lentil beans; another week, brown rice. He would then eat mostly animal foods, at one stretch eating meat two or three times a day.

With each new experiment, he had his blood tested to discover the effects on his cholesterol levels. As he had expected, his cholesterol level rose and fell with his dietary changes. When he included beef and other animal foods, his cholesterol level rose. When he ate plant foods exclusively, his cholesterol fell.

Pritikin was equally diligent about his blood nutrient levels, undergoing regular blood tests to determine if he was experiencing nutrient deficiencies. Contrary to all the warnings, he was never deficient in any vitamin or mineral. After much experimentation, Pritikin finally arrived at a diet made up of brown rice and other whole grains, an abundance of vegetables, beans, and fish. His cholesterol level stabilized at 120 mg/dl and remained there for the rest of his life.

"It really was not that complicated," Pritikin would say many years later. "After a couple of months, I realized I was no different from any of the animal studies. The same way animals drop their cholesterol level, so do humans. I never did run into deficiencies. I was just frightened unnecessarily."

The effects of his diet on his overall health were remarkable. His energy increased dramatically, as did his mental clarity. He went back to work and was more energetic and creative than he had been in decades. It wasn't long before his medical tests confirmed what he had already suspected. In June 1960, just a few months before his forty-fifth birthday, Pritikin underwent a series of tests, including electrocardiogram (EKG), which showed that his heart was getting more blood and, in fact, functioning normally. As his medical record states, he experienced "[d]efinite improvement since the tracing of December 15, 1959 . . . [n]ormal electrocardiogram."

He had cured what his doctors had told him was incurable. But he didn't stop there. Pritikin spent the next twenty-five years using diet and exercise to help tens of thousands of people overcome heart disease, diabetes, high blood pressure, and many other illnesses that to this day have no exclusively pharmaceutical or surgical answer.

Definitive proof that Pritikin's program actually reduced or eliminated the cholesterol plaques in his coronary arteries—and thus reversed coronary heart disease—went unanswered for decades. But forty years later, Dr. Dean Ornish would use virtually the same program as Pritikin to prove that diet and exercise could reverse atherosclerosis in coronary heart disease and thus cure the underlying cause of heart disease, heart attack, and stroke.

DIAGNOSIS, NOT DESTINY

As so many recovery stories have demonstrated, a diagnosis of a serious illness does not necessarily mean the end. Indeed, the power of a medical doctor's prognosis can have a devastating effect on the patient—not so much because doctors have the ability to see the future, but rather because of the titan-like status that society confers on them. Many people see doctors as infallible. But that can be dangerous belief, especially when a doctor gives bad news to a patient.

In his book *Space, Time, and Medicine,* Dr. Larry Dossey tells the story of an old man who turned up at a local hospital emaciated and about to die. Dossey and his fellow physician, a doctor named Jim, performed every test possible on the man, but none revealed a single sign of illness. Finally, Dr. Jim told the man that he was dying. The old man said he already knew that. He also knew why: He had been hexed, he said, by a local shaman. Determined to save his patient's life, Dr. Jim conducted a midnight "de-hexing" ceremony, complete with a candlelight ritual that involved burning a lock of the man's hair. As Dossey put it, "I now realize what I didn't know then.

I was witnessing an archetypal struggle—one shaman battling another shaman—a struggle over life itself."

As it turned out, the ritual worked. The man was convinced that the doctors had succeeded in casting off the curse. The following day, the man was jovial. His appetite returned; he ate copious amounts of food; and soon regained his normal weight. He left the hospital seven days later in joyful spirits and, according to all his tests, in perfectly good health.

For most people today, medical doctors are modern-day shamans. They possess a power to discover illness, destroy it, and save lives. It is an awesome ability, and it explains why doctors are so revered. But when a doctor tells a patient that he or she has only a slim chance of survival, or that he or she is likely about to die, it is often enough to seal that person's fate. I have noticed many times the way a robust man can shrink and wither within weeks of being told he has a terminal illness. Was the sudden progression of the illness merely coincidental with the doctor's statement? Or was the man's demise hastened by the bad news?

The problem for many people who have been diagnosed with serious illnesses is that they must cope with the illnesses as well as the overwhelming feelings that accompany medical prognoses, which, for some amount to a hex. Getting better sometimes means overcoming both the illness and the hex.

It's not surprising, therefore, that many respond to these fears by searching for another authority figure—either another doctor or a complementary healer—who will give them reason to hope and, in effect, remove the hex. Yes, they want effective medicine, to be sure. But most patients have little or no basis to evaluate the medicine apart from what the doctor tells them. And they can believe in the medicine only if the doctor believes in it, too. In effect, the doctor or healer invests his or her personal power and prestige into the remedy so that the patient can believe in it and thus have reason to hope. This is part of the magic behind placebo treatments. But if the doctor does not believe there is much chance of recovery, then what power can the medication possibly have?

AWAKENING THE HEALER WITHIN

Deep within you lies a warrior-healer, an archetype not unlike the Divine Mother, but very different in its content and purpose. The warrior-healer in you, with all its healing power, awakens and engages you in the battle to overcome your illness. Committing your heart and spirit to getting well galvanizes your immune system and healing forces.

The human will to live is a powerful force. By engaging in your own healing treatments and searching for answers, you unleash your own biological, psychological, and spiritual forces that can mean the difference between health and illness, life and death. This is not to say that you will walk the healing path alone. Recovery cannot happen without help from many other people, including doctors, teachers, counselors, guides, and loving supporters. But there is an aspect of the healing process that only you can fulfill, and that work can make all the difference.

In his book, *Love, Medicine, and Miracles,* Dr. Bernie Siegel describes what he calls "exceptional patients" who are often seen by physicians as difficult. Indeed, they do not win popularity contests with doctors. Exceptional patients want to know why tests are done or treatments prescribed. "They're never in their hospital rooms," explains Dr. Siegel.

"Exceptional patients often break the rules," writes Dr. Siegel. They choose treatments according to their own judgment and intuition, often using alternative options in combination with standard medical treatment. Each treatment is evaluated for both its capacity to extend life and enhance the quality of life. Treatments that do not meet these criteria are avoided, while those that are more therapeutic are selected. Exceptional patients also tend to determine for themselves how long they will undergo a given treatment. In short, they are not passive observers. They are involved in every aspect of their healing process. "Exceptional patients are fighters," says Dr. Siegel. "These are the people who very often beat a killer disease."

VIRGINIA'S STORY

Virginia Harper exemplifies Dr. Siegel's description of an exceptional patient. At the age of twenty-two, she was diagnosed with Crohn's disease, an incurable illness that causes the small intestine to become inflamed and ulcerated, resulting in terrible pain, diarrhea, fever, and bloody stools. As treatment, her doctor prescribed anti-inflammatory drugs, which made Virginia bloated and overweight. At the same time, Virginia was also suffering from Takayasu arteritis, a rare and incurable autoimmune condition that causes certain large blood vessels to become inflamed or narrowed, increasing the risk of aneurysm or stroke. The combination of Crohn's disease, Takayasu arteritis, and the medication she was taking produced an array of severe side effects, including intense headaches. Her eyes became sensitive to light. Her joints ached and her feet swelled so severely that she nearly screamed when she placed them on the floor in the morning. Her intestines were a constant source of pain. She was often depressed and weepy. These and other symptoms become even more intense during her many Crohn's flare-ups.

Virginia was told that the disease might be slowed by drug treatment, but that the inflammation could progress through the small intestine and possibly migrate to the large intestine. Many of those suffering from Crohn's require surgery to remove lengths of diseased intestinal tract. In some cases, a colostomy is performed, in which part or all of the large intestine is removed. The end of the intestine is then joined to an opening in the abdomen wall, where a bag is placed to capture waste released from the body.

In Virginia's case, her Crohn's disease was particularly intense and intractable. After two years of medical treatment, her doctor ordered a new regimen of experimental drugs, which he referred to as chemotherapy, but acknowledged that the new treatment was unlikely to bring about any real improvement. In light of this fact, he also suggested she undergo surgery to remove a significant portion of her diseased small intestine. It was then that fate intervened. Virginia's father, an insurance salesman, had met a client who mentioned in passing that his daughter suffered from Takayasu's arteritis, and that her health seemed to improve after she had adopted a diet known as macrobiotics. Virginia's father had to hear more, and after getting all the information he could, drove to Virginia's house, burst into her kitchen, and announced that he had found the answer to both her arteritis and her Crohn's.

Someone else might have reacted skeptically, but for Virginia, everything her father said made perfect sense. Her intestines had to be effected by what she ate, Virginia realized. Her diet was atrocious by any standard. Fast food, junk food, greasy meats, fat-laden snacks, chips of all kinds, candy, cookies, chocolate, soda—these were among her staples. At the age of twenty-four, Virginia stood five feet three inches tall and was forty pounds overweight. Her food choices were affecting every aspect of her health.

Her father had already found a macrobiotic counselor, Bill Spear, in Connecticut, whom Virginia contacted immediately and arranged to meet. Bill Spear would guide her for the next two years, but it only took a month before she felt improvements in her condition. Within weeks of changing her food, Virginia experienced less intestinal pain, gas, bloating, and swelling of her feet. These signs were small, she acknowledged, but she felt certain that they were the consequence of her change in diet.

Virginia had not yet begun the new drug regimen, and her date for surgery was now approaching. She met with her doctor and cautiously informed him that she had changed her diet and now wanted to postpone both the drugs and the operation.

"How have you been feeling?" her doctor asked her.

"Very good," she said. "I really do feel much better."

"Oh? Well, that's great," the doctor said. "Have you experienced any changes in your condition since we last saw each other?"

"Well, that's what I want to talk to you about. I want to postpone the chemotherapy and the surgery," Virginia told him.

"Why?" he asked. Virginia could hear alarm rising in his voice.

"Because I have started a macrobiotic diet and I want to give it some more time to see if it could make me well," Virginia answered. "I've already experienced some small signs that it's helping me."

"You can't do that," the doctor demanded. He then got up from behind his desk and started toward Virginia, who was sitting in a chair opposite his desk. "That food is going to be too hard on you. You're going to hurt yourself. There's not one bit of scientific proof that a macrobiotic diet can do any good."

"How is it going to hurt me?" Virginia asked him.

"As your doctor I can't allow it. You are in a very delicate condition and that crazy diet can only do you harm."

"I have already been doing it and it's helping me some. I want to give it more time," Virginia responded, emotion rising in her voice now.

"You cannot go on a macrobiotic diet," the doctor confidently asserted. "It's crazy and dangerous. You cannot follow a diet like that. I will not go on treating you if you do."

Virginia broke down in tears and told him flatly, "This is my only hope. I need you to support me. This diet makes sense. The food is going into my intestines. That's where the problem is. Look at me. I'm twenty-four years old. If I make it to thirty, I'm not going to have my intestines. This is my last chance and I need you to help me."

Shocked by Virginia's reaction, and perhaps a bit chastened, her doctor relented and agreed to monitor her, but only if she saw him more often. She agreed. Over the course of the next year, Virginia's condition steadily improved until, much to her doctor's surprise, she was pronounced free of all Crohn's-related symptoms. She lost weight, weaned herself off all her medications, and regained her life. She also experienced a complete elimination of all signs and symptoms of Takayasu arteritis. Her medical tests confirmed her daily experience. Doctors could find no signs of either Crohn's disease or Takayasu arteritis.

At the time of this writing, Virginia is still free of any symptoms or signs of Crohn's disease. She is in excellent health and lives an extremely active life, which includes teaching people how to overcome Crohn's and other inflammatory bowel disorders.

MAKING YOUR OWN DECISIONS

Like Nathan Pritikin, Virginia made a choice. She did not accept an exclusively medical approach to her illness, even when her doctor attempted to impose his authority on her. But nothing the doctor had suggested was working. On the contrary, even while being treated, she suffered ongoing symptoms and regular flare-ups, many of which forced her to be hospitalized.

Her life was literally being destroyed by the disease. Immediately upon hearing about macrobiotics, she began studying the diet, the effects of plant food on her digestion, and what intestines need to function properly. As she learned more, her trust and intuition led her to make an even deeper commitment to her healing path. Indeed, Virginia realized that only a full commitment would be enough to give her a chance at healing. If she were willing to make that commitment, she realized, it might work, and it did.

At the core of Virginia's healing journey is a question that she had to ask herself: Who is ultimately responsible for my health, me or my doctor? The answer seems obvious, but all too many of us surrender control of our choices and responsibilities to authority figures, including doctors. And with that surrender, we can easily find ourselves saying yes to medical options that we did not feel entirely comfortable with, or, perhaps knew in our hearts that we were better off avoiding.

In addition, people who surrender control of their medical choices often are reluctant to explore complementary alternatives, in part because their doctors dismiss such practices as worthless or even dangerous. In such cases, a patient can sometimes adopt the biases of his or her doctor without ever knowing if a particular form of complementary care could be helpful. One woman I recently worked with confided in me that she was afraid of adopting any complementary healing methods because she feared she might offender her doctor.

Fortunately, the medical landscape has changed over the last three decades. Many forms of complementary treatment have not only been proven safe but also highly effective at supporting the body's underlying healing forces. To be sure, medical doctors are an essential part of your treatment, but they are not the only part.

Both Virginia and Nathan remained in close contact with their doctors, who performed regular diagnostic tests to monitor their health statuses. If the diets they chose to follow had had no therapeutic value, or had actually made their diseases worse, the medical tests would have revealed them to be harmful. As it happened, medical tests showed that the two were able to make steady improvement. Both Nathan and Virginia found their doctors were essential sources of medical information and advice. Neither Virginia nor Nathan had any interest in pursuing a fantasy or proving an ideological point about diet and health; all they wanted was to get better. If a particular program didn't work, both wanted to be rid of it as quickly as possible. In both cases, doctors were there to provide medical information and help them make wise decisions.

TAKING YOUR OWN APPROACH

Make medicine work for you. People oftentimes say that their doctors work for them, but how many truly feel they have hired their physicians and are really in control of their medical decisions? Most people become passive, powerless patients. They go to hospitals or their doctors' offices and then wait to be seen. They submit to the tests these doctors order. They accept the medications or chemotherapy that they prescribe, often without question, and take such drugs for as long as they are recommended. They undergo the surgeries that their doctors say are needed. They comply with their doctors' orders. The patient is not in control; the doctor is. Many doctors are so used to being in charge that they become irate, as Virginia Harper's doctor did, when a patient decides to adopt a healing approach that is not included in the doctor's conventional arsenal. Conflicts such as these are not inevitable, but they are common, especially when a patient realizes that it is his or her life on the line, and that, in the end, it is his or her responsibility to make the important decisions.

There are doctors who welcome the moment their patients become co-healers, but these patients may not know it until they explore complementary healing methods and share them with their physicians. For many people, wanting a degree of control over the healing process may seem like pure hubris, but science has shown that patients who exert some control over their circumstances experience a significant improvement in immune function. On the other hand, those who experience helplessness are more likely to suffer significant declines in immune strength.

A study done by Yale researchers William J. Sieber and Judith Rodin explored the physiological effects of prolonged stress, which in this case took the form of noise levels. Sieber and Rodin examined two groups of people: one group that could control noise levels, and another group that could not. The researchers found that the group that could control the noise experienced no significant drop in immune reaction. The group that could not control the noise, however, suffered sharp declines in natural killer cell activity—a specific type of immune cell that attacks and destroys bacteria, viruses, and cancer cells.

Animal studies have shown that the ability to exert control over one's environment plays a crucial role in health. A study published in *Science* compared two groups of laboratory animals, both of which were subjected to unexpected and repeated shock. One group was able to escape the shock, while the other was not able to do so. The scientists found that the group that was able to escape the shock experienced little or no impairment of their immune systems, but the animals that had no control over the stress of their circumstances experienced significant declines in immunity and greater susceptibility to disease.

Taking control of your situation, even in small ways, can have a profound impact on your outlook, hope, and immune function. What's more, the benefits of taking control can build over time. As you go deeper into the healing process and find tools that independently improve your health, your feelings of control—and with them your immune response—can grow even stronger.

DOES TAKING RESPONSIBILITY MEAN YOU ARE TO BLAME?

Several years ago, a woman asked me for advice on how she might support her own recovery from breast cancer. I suggested dietary and lifestyle changes. Weeks later, I asked if she had made any progress after incorporating those changes. "No," she said. "I decided that I could not change my way of eating because if I did that, I would be admitting that I had created my cancer. I can't do that," she said. "I don't want to feel that I'm to blame for my illness."

I couldn't help but sympathize. Many people confuse the act of taking responsibility with blaming themselves for their past actions and perceived mistakes. The truth is that no one can be blamed for becoming ill. Illness is caused by too many variables over which we have little or no control—genetics, for example, or childhood exposure to certain harmful environmental substances. In addition, all of us have been subjected to varying degrees of psychological trauma, which can impair immune function and predispose us to illness. For virtually all of us, emotional pain drives our food and lifestyle choices, which result in health issues for many.

Even relationships with parents can play a crucial role in our long-term health. A long-term study conducted by Harvard University researchers on male students who graduated from Harvard between 1939 and 1944 found that warm relationships, especially with mother, were pivotal in determining a person's health and success in life. The study, known as the Grant Study, followed 268 healthy students for up to 75 years. Among its most important findings was the fact that 91 percent of study participants who said that they did not have warm, loving relationships with their parents, especially with mother, were later diagnosed with serious illnesses, including heart disease, high blood pressure, ulcers, dementia, and alcoholism.

Conversely, only 45 percent of the former students who had reported positive relationships with their parents, especially with their mothers, were later diagnosed with serious diseases. In short, those who had warm relationships with their mothers had half the rates of illness that those who described their relationships with their mothers as cold or difficult.

Of course, not everyone who gets sick necessarily has a poor relationship with his or her parents, but the study does suggest that early life experiences can be a factor in determining health. Combine the Harvard study with the reality that many people are exposed to disease-promoting substances throughout life via experiences over which they have little control and you may begin to see how irrelevant self-blame is in the expression of disease.

Among the keys to dissolving self-blame is compassion for all that you are experiencing and, indeed, for what other people suffer in life. Among the more interesting realities that we learn on this path is that self-blame, guilt, and shame cannot be sustained in the face of compassion for self and others. Compassion dissolves all forms of judgment. This is the moment when the mother archetype, the Divine Mother consciousness, informs you that blame of yourself or others is based on an incomplete picture of reality, and that factors both outside your control and beyond your awareness played essential roles in the creation of your current circumstances.

What matters is what you do now. And from this point onward, much can be done to strengthen your immune system and healing forces. As you will see in much greater detail later on, there is a sleeping giant within you that, once aroused, can turn the tide in your favor. Only by taking control of your healing process, which is to say, becoming fully engaged and responsible for your own recovery, can these powerful healing forces be awakened and launched against illness.

THE HEALING POWER OF PURE HONESTY

In the early stages of the healing process, certain characteristics emerge as essential. Among them is the willingness to be deeply honest with yourself and to search your soul for your own inner truth. Another is pure courage, especially in the face of new information that you feel intuitively is important to your healing. Nathan Pritikin happened to stumble across a series of obscure scientific studies that examined the effects of food rationing on European populations during World War II, but his discovery would have been meaningless were it not for his honest appraisal of his own eating habits and his courageous willingness to change his own behavior in light of new information that had presented itself.

Virginia Harper's life would have been very different had it not been for her willingness to listen with an open mind and an open heart to her father's sudden and unexpected encounter with someone who knew about Takayasu arteritis and had been using a strange-sounding plant-based diet called macrobiotics. Not only did Virginia listen, but she also acted with great honesty, courage, and intelligence on the information she received. Taking responsibility for your recovery means more than merely gaining information. It also means being willing to change—indeed, evolve—on the basis of the information you obtain.

Nevertheless, not all the information you come across along your healing path will be worth pursuing. Many claims made about health programs prove to be worthless in the end. Being responsible means looking carefully at each medical or complementary approach being offered to you. It means studying the approach and learning to feel and be guided by your judgment and subtle intuitive wisdom. In time, you will develop trusting relationships with medical doctors and holistic healers and guides who can help you make wise decisions. But in the end, every decision must finally be your own. It is the only way to be truly at peace with your healing path.

WHAT TO DO NOW

The following guidance will help you start the process of gaining vital information, as well as applying it to your own circumstance. These are some of the actions you can take right now.

Learn More about Your Illness

There are several different categories of information that you will need to gather at this point. Some of it must be a purely medical, scientific understanding of your illness and the types of medical approaches used to treat your disease. It's important to have an understanding of as many medical options as are available to you. Much of the information you will require will be available in books, on websites, and in articles on your illness. The Resources section of this book (see page 217) can direct you to different sources of information—from medical and scientific research to sources of holistic and complementary healing.

While there are many different websites for orthodox medical information, good places to start your search include the Mayo Clinic (www.mayoclinic.org). One of the leading hospitals and research centers in the world, it offers an online service that provides medical information on virtually every medical condition, along with books and articles on medical treatment and wellness. The Cleveland Clinic (www.clevelanclinic.org) is another of the world's leading hospitals and research centers. Its website provides more than 5,000 articles, videos, and podcasts to the general public on diseases, disorders, and medical treatments. The Cleveland Clinic also provides a health information specialist to help you search the Clinic's library and find information you need.

The National Institutes of Health website offers a wide menu of information on diseases, medical treatments, scientific studies, guidance for finding medical care and for communicating effectively with your doctor. In addition, the NIH offers the National Institutes of Health online library, PubMed (www.pubmed.gov). You can use the NIH library to look up individual studies on any medical or scientific health-related question. It is an enormous and extremely valuable resource. A good website for introductory information is WebMD (www.webmd.com), which provides basic, easily accessible information on virtually all illnesses and disorders. Finally, Google Scholar (scholar.google.com) is another excellent resource for scientific studies on any medical question.

Speak Openly to Your Doctor

It is essential to speak openly to your doctor and get all the information you need to make informed decisions about your medical care. Questions you should ask your doctor include the following:

- What is the proposed treatment attempting to accomplish, and how will it do that?

- Does this treatment offer the possibility of a cure?

- Is there a survival benefit to this treatment? In other words, will I live longer if I undergo this treatment?

- What percentage of people with my illness who undergo this particular medical treatment experience longer life?

- On average, how long is life extended for those who undergo this treatment?

- What are the possible side effects of this treatment? Do those side effects include death?

- What should I expect regarding the quality of my life during and after the treatment period?

- What does the science show for those who avoid treatment entirely?

After you have asked these questions, you will want to spend some time reflecting on a question that only you can answer: Do the potential risks outweigh the potential benefits of this treatment? You must decide whether this treatment is the right choice for you. Listen to your gut.

Assess Health Patterns

The most common characteristic shared by those who recover from illness is the ability to assess dietary choices, exercise patterns, stress levels, emotional patterns, relationships, and lifestyle habits on an ongoing basis. Once they see their imbalances, they make important changes and adjustments to their behaviors that positively affect their health statuses.

For now, answer the questions below as honestly as you can. Doing so will help you prepare for the kinds of changes you will want to make as you progress through the rest of this book. Ask yourself the following:

- Do my eating habits and lifestyle support recovery? Are there changes in my eating habits or daily patterns that could be made to strengthen my chances of recovery? What am I doing to learn more about the relationship between diet and health? Am I prepared to change my way of eating to support my recovery?

- Are my stress levels too high? (Much of your stress may be coming from your illness, but ask yourself if there are stressors other than your illness that you could manage better or even eliminate.) What is my relationship with time? Am I continually short of time? If so, why? What must I do to change my life so that I have more time and less stress?

■ Do I exercise enough? If not, what can I do today to start exercising? Can I take a daily walk, even if it's for only ten minutes?

■ Am I getting the love I need? Am I giving love to those I truly care about? What can I do now to enhance my life in both of these areas?

■ Am I in conflict with the people I love or are my important relationships at peace? What are the sources of that conflict? What can I do to resolve that conflict so that I can be more at peace with myself and those I love? Whom do I need to forgive? Am I actively involved in forgiving those I love? Do I need to ask for forgiveness? What is holding me back from doing so?

■ Is my work helping or hindering my healing now? Is it taking too much of my time and energy? Does my gut intuition tell me that I should leave my job, if only temporarily?

■ What is my relationship with the spiritual dimension of my life? Am I at peace with God? Are there practices I could do to create a better relationship with my perception of the Divine? What can I do today that will create greater spiritual peace in my life?

Where to Start

The Resources section (see page 217) of this book will help you find sources of credible scientific information, as well as medical doctors, scientists, and healers who can help you gather the highest quality cutting edge approaches to healing. Among the people you should turn to immediately for the information you seek include the following:

■ T. Colin Campbell, PhD, director of the Center for Nutrition Studies and professor emeritus of Nutritional Biochemistry at Cornell University. Dr. Campbell is coauthor of *The China Study* and the lead scientist on the landmark research known as the China Study.

■ Caldwell Esselstyn, MD, surgeon and former President of the Staff of the Cleveland Clinic, Lyndhurst, Ohio. He is the author of *Prevent and Reverse Heart Disease.*

- John McDougall, MD, founder of Doctor McDougall's Medical Center in Santa Rosa, California. Dr. McDougall is the author of several books, including *The Starch Solution*.

- The Pritikin Longevity Center and Resort, Miami, Florida. The Pritikin Longevity Center provides residential and medical care for its diet, exercise, and lifestyle program.

Other highly qualified sources of complementary care are also provided in the Resources section.

Regularly Monitor Your Condition

You will want to monitor your health and progress through both objective and subjective methods. The objective methods are your medical tests and physician's assessments. Ask your doctor which tests represent the key biomedical markers for health and illness. In the next chapter, some of the most important objective tests will be identified for you. You will also want to keep track of your medications and their dosages, especially as they can change over time.

Subjective measures are largely based on how you feel. It's important to keep a record of any symptoms you may have, the intensity of those symptoms, and your energy levels, moods, and outlook. It's also important to be able to track how complementary healing methods, as well as changes in diet and lifestyle, affect your subjective states. For that, I recommend a healing journal in which you record, as frequently as possible, both your objective and subjective assessments.

Join Support Groups

Most cities and local communities provide support groups for virtually all common health challenges. People in these groups exchange vital information and personal experiences with medical and complementary care. Local people can provide referrals for doctors, nurses, and complementary practitioners of almost every type. People in support groups will not only share information but also compassionate support, simply because many of them understand what you are going through as few others can. Support groups are one the most important sources of guidance, care, and practical information.

In addition to in-person support meetings, there are many online support groups that can provide essential information on medical and complementary care. You can use any search engine to find support groups for specific health issues. You can also use facebook to search for and become a member of support groups of all types.

As your knowledge and compassion grow, so will your confidence and personal power. Your newfound confidence will likely encourage you to assume a more powerful role in your treatment program. You will then realize that you have entered a new phase of your healing process, one that is driven by your need to adopt practical behaviors that promote your own healing forces. At that point, you will be ready for the third step of your journey.

$\mathcal{A}$DOPT
A HEALING DIET

A lover of steaks, hamburgers, French fries, and milk shakes, former US president Bill Clinton was once known as a junk food junky. While following Clinton on the campaign trail for the White House, a CNN reporter watched Clinton buy a box of doughnuts and proceed to eat every one of them. Not surprisingly, Clinton had a long history of health problems, most notably advanced heart disease. In 2004, he had quadruple coronary bypass surgery. In 2011, he had another operation to insert two stents placed in a coronary artery that had become blocked. He also suffered from weight problems, at one point getting up as high as 236 pounds.

Things were not looking good, Clinton admitted, and he wondered if he would live long enough to see his daughter married and have children. That's when he decided to change his way of eating. In an interview, Clinton said, "I wanted to live to be a grandfather, so I decided to pick the diet that I thought would maximize my chances of long-term survival." Clinton adopted a vegan diet, eschewing meat, dairy products, eggs, and anything else derived from an animal. Clinton went on to lose thirty pounds and now says he feels great.

"[My doctor] asked me to eat organic salmon once a week," he told CNN. "I do, but I'd just as soon be without it. The vegan diet is what I like the best. . . . I have more energy. . . . For me the no dairy thing, because I had an allergy, has really helped a lot. And I feel good." Meanwhile, his heart has made a remarkable recovery. His daughter, Chelsea, said that her father's doctor tells him that his heart is actually stronger than it was ten years ago. "I'm trying to be one of those experimenters," Clinton said. "Since 1986, several hundred people who have tried essentially a plant-based diet—not ingesting any cholesterol from any source—have seen their bodies start to heal themselves; break up the arterial blockage, break up the calcium deposits around the heart. Eighty-two percent of people who have done this have had the result, so I want to see if I can be one of them."

Heart disease is the number one killer in the Western world, but a plant-based diet can have a profound effect on one's recovery process. According to Bill Clinton, his vegan diet is the reason his heart troubles are a thing of the past. "I might not be around if I hadn't become a vegan," he said.

COMMON FACTORS

Health authorities and the media have led us to believe that illnesses such as heart disease, high blood pressure, type-2 diabetes, and certain forms of cancer are very different diseases and therefore arise from very different causes. But in the great majority of cases, these illnesses are, in fact, different manifestations of the same underlying factors: high insulin levels, high levels of inflammation, and being overweight. This underlying disease state is the true basis of most of the health epidemics that afflict and kill us today, and the single greatest contributor to this state is the type of diet most people eat today.

Insulin Resistance

Insulin is a hormone that opens cells so that blood sugar, or glucose, can enter and be utilized as fuel. Insulin is essential to life—without fuel the body dies. The problem is that too much fuel and too much insulin can be disastrous. When insulin and blood sugar become elevated and stay elevated over time, health problems follow.

Cells can absorb only so much glucose. When too much glucose continues to pour into the bloodstream, the body creates more insulin in order to force the excess glucose into cells. Under such conditions, cells are overwhelmed by the high glucose and insulin levels and begin to deny entry to glucose altogether, creating a condition known as insulin resistance. Insulin resistance is the basis of type-2 diabetes—the form of diabetes in which glucose metabolism malfunctions and the person produces more insulin than is healthy.

In a high-insulin environment, glucose is converted into fat, causing rapid weight gain. Many overweight people try to limit their calories, but when insulin is high the body continues converting available glucose into fat and thus causes ever-expanding weight gain. Globules of fat known as triglycerides pour into the bloodstream and cut off oxygen to cells, killing some, deforming others, and increasing the risks of heart attack, stroke, and cancer.

Contrary to popular belief, fat cells are extremely active. As Dr. Pinchas Cohen, pediatric endocrinologist at UCLA Medical Center in Santa Monica, has said, "There are lots of products going out of them, and most of them are bad." Among the harmful substances produced by fat are interleukin-6 (Il-6) and tumor necrosis factor (TNF), both of which are highly inflammatory. They also produce estrogens, the female hormone that plays a major role in the onset of cancers of the breast, ovarian, uterine, and prostate. All of which explains why being overweight is recognized as a leading risk factor in cancer.

In a 2003 study published in the *New England Journal of Medicine*, researchers reported that being overweight drives up your chances of contracting cancers of the lymph system, kidneys, liver, gall bladder, pancreas, breast, uterus, ovaries, cervix, prostate, colon, rectum, and stomach. Moreover, the *Journal of the National Cancer Institute* found that overweight and obese women are twice as likely to contract breast cancer as women who are at their ideal weight.

The body's attempts to force glucose into cells can result in injury to these cells. As cells resist, these injuries multiply, causing immune cells to arrive on the scene in order to deal with possible infection. These immune cells trigger an inflammatory reaction within the body, which causes further cellular injury, including damage to DNA. Many cells die, but others can become malignant and thus cancerous. It is also important to note that insulin is a mitogen, meaning it stimulates cells to multiply. Once cancer has taken hold in the system, high insulin levels serve as fuel for cancer's growth and proliferation.

What Raises Insulin?

Insulin levels rise when you begin to exercise, are under stress, or eat carbohydrate-rich food. During exercise, your body releases additional fuel into your bloodstream and, at the same time, produces more insulin so that this fuel can be utilized by your cells. As you continue to exercise, however, glucose is essentially burned off, and both glucose and insulin start to fall into healthy ranges. They will stay there as long as you exercise regularly and maintain a healthy diet. So, exercise is ultimately an effective way to lower both blood sugar and insulin, but the powerful benefits of lower insulin may be experienced only if exercise is accompanied by a healing, plant-based diet.

Stress triggers the "flight or fight" response, which produces a boost of energy to prime the body to run away from perceived danger or tackle it head on, whether that danger is real or not. This reaction is understandably associated with elevations in glucose and insulin. If a stressful event is followed by exercise—a walk, for example—the excess glucose and insulin can be burned off. But if stress is chronic and exercise is avoided, insulin and glucose levels can remain high and trigger the kinds of harmful biochemical conditions previously described.

During digestion, carbohydrates are converted into glucose, raising insulin levels. But not all carbs are created equal. Some are good and offer health benefits, while others are bad and downright unnatural. Arguably, bad carbs should be considered products of factories rather than nature. They've been stripped of much of their nutrition and fiber during processing. The long, complex carbohydrate chains that nature arranged for them have been shattered. Without their fiber content and complex carbohydrate chains, these carbs are now simple sugars, able to be absorbed into the bloodstream almost instantly. This immediate absorption causes a flood of glucose in the bloodstream, which spikes insulin levels.

If processed foods, rich in their simple sugars, are eaten consistently—which is the case for most people in the modern world today—all the dangerous conditions associated with high glucose and high insulin are set in motion. Thankfully, sources of bad carbs are easy to spot. Many of them are white foods: refined sugar, white bread, white rolls, pastries, bagels, and baguettes. Bad carbs are also found in candy, soda pop, energy drinks, breakfast cereals, and most snacks, including pretzels and potato chips.

Good carbs, on the other hand, cause only moderate elevations in glucose and insulin levels. They are also good sources of plant-based nutrients, energy, and fiber. Good carbs are bound together in long, complex carbohydrate chains that must be acted upon by your intestines in order to release the individual carbohydrates into your bloodstream. Good carbs are also trapped in the fiber of food and thus require additional work by your gut to be freed and then absorbed by your cells. These freed sugars are dripped into your bloodstream, giving you hours of sustained energy. There is no sudden flooding of your bloodstream with glucose, no insulin spike, only the slow release of fuel into your system.

Sources of good carbs are whole, unprocessed plant foods, including nearly all vegetables and some fruits, which help keep insulin levels low. Whole grains such as quinoa, amaranth, and brown rice also have moderate effects on insulin levels and so are also good choices.

By choosing good carbs, you will keep your insulin levels low. Lowering your insulin with healing foods will also dramatically reduce inflammation, cause you to lose weight, and boost your entire health-restoring system. The changes can help you overcome serious illness and get well.

The Glycemic Index

The glycemic index reveals the relative effects of individual foods on blood sugar and insulin levels. The following list divides a number of common foods into two categories according to their effects on insulin.

Low-glycemic foods are those that cause only small elevations in insulin and thus provide all the benefits of a low-insulin diet.

Foods that stimulate a significant rise in insulin are designated high-glycemic foods. These cause weight gain easily and, if consumed regularly, can lead to all the disorders associated with insulin resistance.

In general, unprocessed plant foods are low on the glycemic index, while processed foods tend to be high on the glycemic index.

LOW-GLYCEMIC FOODS				
VEGETABLES AND ROOTS	**FRUIT**	**BEANS AND LEGUMES**	**WHOLE GRAINS**	**PROCESSED FOODS**
Bok Choy	Apples	Aduki beans	Barley, pearled	Fettuccine, white
Broccoli	Apricots	Black beans	Brown rice	Spaghetti, white
Cabbage	Bananas	Black-eyed beans	Rye	Spaghetti, whole wheat
Carrots	Cherries	Chickpeas		Whole-grain bread
Cauliflower	Grapefruit	Kidney beans		
Celery	Grapes	Lentils		
Collard greens	Kiwi	Peas		
Cucumber	Oranges	Soy beans		
Kale	Peaches			
Leafy greens	Pears			
Spinach	Plums			
Sweet potatoes	Tomato			
Yams				

Both white fettuccine and white spaghetti are composed chiefly of complex carbohydrates and are more slowly absorbed than other processed foods such as bagels, baguettes, or pastries. Whole-grain spaghetti is even lower on the glycemic index than its white counterpart, but not by much. Both whole-grain spaghetti and white spaghetti and fettuccine are considered low-glycemic foods.

HIGH-GLYCEMIC FOODS				
BREADS AND FLOUR PRODUCTS	**VEGETABLES**	**FRUIT**	**SNACKS AND DESSERTS**	
Baguette	Parsnips, baked	Dates	Cakes	Jams
Breakfast cereals	Potato		Candies	Jellies
Waffles			Cookies	Potato chips
White bread			Corn Chips	Pretzels
White Rice			Cupcakes	Pudding
White rolls			Doughnuts	Soda

Inflammation

Inflammation may be the most common factor behind most degenerative diseases today. Inflammation occurs whenever your immune system reacts to any kind of threat to your health, whether it is a bacterial infection, virus, diseased cells, or the presence of harmful contaminants in your air, food, or water. Your immune system quickly identifies the troublesome agent that has entered your system and neutralizes it in relatively short time. Once the threat has passed, your immune system stands down and returns to a state of quiet alertness, ready to pounce when the next invader appears. This happens day after day, year after year, throughout most of your life, without you ever taking notice of the miracles occurring within you.

Unfortunately, as powerful as the immune system is, it has its limits. The challenge it faces is not unlike that faced by a circus juggler. Keep throwing bowling pins at the juggler and eventually, no matter how good he is, he is going to falter and drop the pins. Essentially, this is what can happen to the immune system. It can become overwhelmed by the presence of too many varied threats to health. The immune system can easily find itself battling an endless array of pathogens, environmental contaminants, harmful dietary substances, the consequences of high insulin, and the dangerous chemicals produced by chronic stress and excess body fat.

In order to deal with these many dangers, the immune system produces oxidants—highly reactive oxygen molecules—that, like guided missiles, are fired at cancer cells, bacteria, or viruses. The system also produces antibodies, which have the power to neutralize diseased cells and pathogens. These antibodies are enhanced by what is known as the complement system, which boosts the ability of antibodies to get rid of damaged cells. These and other weapons in the immune system's arsenal are highly effective. But in a polluted biochemistry, the battles become too many, and inevitably there is collateral damage. Healthy cells are attacked in addition to diseased cells. Some are destroyed, while others are damaged.

As famed surgeon and television show host Dr. Mehmet Oz once told me in an interview, "Inflammation is really the destruction of the body by friendly fire. Our own immune system is turned against us, which is pretty scary when you realize just how powerful that system is."

Scientists now recognize inflammation as one of the primary causes of life-threatening illness. "The current theory is that low-grade, sub-acute inflammation—that is to say, inflammation that does not manifest overt symptoms—can lead to an increased risk of heart disease, cancer, diabetes, obesity and other illnesses," said Dr. Michael Wargovich, one of the nation's top cancer researchers. "Among the causes of inflammation is our culture's diet, which contains many pro-inflammatory foods." The fact is that when immune cells are forced to deal with too many harmful substances, inflammation rages, and illness tends to follow.

The two leading killer diseases, heart disease and cancer, demonstrate the terrible consequences that can arise when the immune system is confronted with too much saturated fat, which generally comes from consumption of too many animal products. Saturated fat is converted into blood cholesterol by the liver, specifically a type of cholesterol called LDL (low-density lipoprotein) cholesterol, which is often referred to as "bad cholesterol." Once in your bloodstream, LDL particles infiltrate the inner lining of your arteries, which then oxidize or decay. This situation is then seen by the immune system as a threat to health. Macrophages, a type of immune cell, come bounding down on the LDL and essentially gobble them up. These immune cells become bloated and sick as a result of high levels of LDL, a condition that triggers an even bigger immune reaction that takes place within your artery walls. In other words, the war continues in your arteries.

Eventually, your artery walls will become thick, hard, and swollen with immune cells bloated with LDL. Soon, masses of boils pop up within arterial passageways in a condition known as atherosclerosis. These boils are highly unstable and prone to rupture, and when they do, they open a wound inside the artery wall. Clotting proteins rush to the scene and form a scab-like clot, or thrombus, over the wound, but as ruptures continue, these clots are set free and float downstream. They may be too big to pass through narrow openings in arteries and thus can block blood supply to the heart or brain, causing a heart attack or stroke.

"The research has . . . established a key role for inflammation in atherosclerosis," states Peter Libby in the May 2002 issue of *Scientific American.* "This process—the same one that causes infected cuts to become red, swollen, hot and painful—underlies all phases of the disorder, from the creation of plaques to their growth and rupture. . . ."

Animal fat also seems to play a key role in the inflammatory process that leads to cancer. As inflammation mounts, free radicals multiply and attack your cells, bombarding cell membranes and even DNA, the brain center of cells. Under such a barrage, most cells die, but some can become cancerous. Researchers have consistently found that the higher levels of saturated fat in the diet, the higher the risk of cancer.

Scientists at Harvard Medical School followed 90,655 premenopausal women, all between the ages of twenty-six and forty-six, for eight years, monitoring their diets, lifestyles, and disease patterns. The researchers found that those women whose diets were composed of the most animal foods—especially animal fats—had the highest levels of cancer. The study leader, epidemiologist Dr. Euryoung Cho, was quoted as saying, "Cooked red meat contains carcinogens, and high-fat dairy products contain fat-soluble hormones that may increase risk" of breast cancer. When asked by WebMD about the Harvard study, Dr. Otis Brawley, associate director of Winship Cancer Institute at Emory University School of Medicine in Atlanta, said, "Believe it. . . . [Consumption of animal fat] makes enough difference that it matters. This study is not definitive; it is highly, highly suggestive that it's best to stay away from animal fat."

Overweight

In light of all the social pressures, weight loss is usually seen through an aesthetic lens more than for its positive effects on health. But the evidence is overwhelming that weight loss is one of the most powerful steps you can take in the treatment of disease. As proof, consider one of the body's biochemical heroes, adiponectin.

When you start to lose weight, your fat cells cease producing harmful substances and instead secrete a protein called adiponectin, which many scientists now see as a game changer when it comes to dealing with disease.

Indeed, no drug yet created comes close to having the range of positive effects that adiponectin has on the body and the healing process. It is highly anti-inflammatory. It cools the immune response and lowers levels of free radicals throughout the body, especially in diseased areas where inflammation is most concentrated. It restores insulin sensitivity and reduces insulin resistance. In fact, some studies have shown that when weight loss is accelerated, the sudden rise of adiponectin is powerful enough to take people out of insulin resistance. It sends out chemical messengers that tell the body to clear inflammatory chemicals from a specific area, thereby reducing the amount of toxicity in areas where disease is proliferating. It triggers anti-angiogenesis, meaning it blocks blood flow to tumors, thus depriving cancerous cells from life-giving oxygen and nutrients. In other words, it suffocates and starves tumors. Finally, it induces apoptosis, or programmed cell death, in cancer cells.

Many doctors urge cancer patients to avoid weight loss, but research clearly shows that when cancer patients adopt a plant-based diet and lose weight, they experience a decrease in the production of inflammatory compounds and an increase in adiponectin, both of which are associated with longer life.

WHAT TO AVOID

For those dealing with a serious illness, certain foods and food constituents should be avoided. Among the most troublesome are dairy products, processed foods, trans fatty acids, vegetable oils that oxidize at low temperatures, and synthetic additives. Excessive intake of animal protein is also discouraged.

You may be surprised to see protein and dairy products on the list, as they have long been considered healthy choices, but that belief has come more from effective marketing than from science. Researchers have known for decades that excess protein is harmful to health, as is consumption of products made from cow's milk.

During digestion of animal protein, an amino acid called methionine is metabolized into a substance called homocysteine, which acts like battery acid on the walls of the arteries, creating open wounds in arterial tissue and triggering an inflammatory process.

"The inside lining of the artery is like Teflon," Dr. Oz said. "It creates a smooth surface so that blood can easily pass through the artery. Homocysteine burns away some of that surface to expose the medial layer below the

Teflon coating. Once it's exposed, it attracts more LDL particles and immune cells. That medial layer is electrically charged. So the result is something like a thunderstorm inside your arteries."

This thunderstorm, with its electrical bursts, injures the arteries' Teflon-like coating all the more, thus creating more wounds, which lead to more inflammation and atherosclerotic plaques. As if that were not enough, homocysteine also boosts the formation of blood clots, increasing the size of plaques and elevating risks of heart attack and stroke. The body attempts to protect itself from these events by utilizing folic acid (also known as folate or vitamin B_9), vitamin B_6, and vitamin B_{12} to convert homocysteine into a harmless substance. Folic acid and vitamin B_6 come from plant sources, especially green vegetables and beans. Vitamin B_{12} comes from bacteria on plant foods eaten by animals and tends to accumulate in animal sources of food, including in fish. People on a high-protein, low-plant diet are often low in folate and B_6, and consequently are at greater risk of heart disease.

Milk and milk products are harmful to health in a number of ways. First, whole milk and whole-milk products contain saturated fats, and therefore can be especially dangerous to those facing serious illness. Milk, cheese, and yogurt have been shown to increase blood levels of a compound known as insulin-like growth factor (IGF-1), which has been associated with the onset and growth of cancer, especially cancers of the breast and prostate. A study published in *Science* showed that men with the highest levels of IGF-1 had four times the risk of prostate cancer than men with the lowest levels of IGF-1. This same trend exists for women, as those with high levels of IGF-1 have been linked to an increased rate of breast cancer. In his book *Eat, Drink, and Be Healthy,* Harvard Medical School Dean of Nutrition Dr. Walter Willett states, "In nine separate studies, the strongest and most consistent dietary factor linked with prostate cancer was high consumption of milk or dairy products. In the largest of these, the Health Professionals Follow-up Study, men who drank two or more glasses of milk a day were almost twice as likely to develop advanced or metastatic (spreading) prostate cancer as those who didn't drink milk at all."

Concerns have been raised about milk's possible link to other types of cancers as well. Dr. Willett points to earlier research done at Harvard University by Dr. Daniel Cramer. Dr. Cramer found that, once in the body, the sugar in dairy products, known as lactose, is converted into another form of sugar called galactose. Galactose is broken down by enzymes produced by the liver. When the body's ability to break down galactose is exceeded, these sugars build up and in women can damage their ovaries. Women who have low levels of the enzyme needed to break down galactose are three times more likely to suffer ovarian cancer than women who have normal levels of this enzyme.

Milk products, like all animal products, are high in protein, especially sulfur amino acids, which increase acid levels in the blood and leach calcium from bones, according to a report published in *Dietitian's Edge*. According to Dr. Belinda S. O'Connell, "We know that dietary protein intake influences urinary calcium losses with each gram of dietary protein, increasing urinary calcium losses by 1-1.5 mg. This means that a person who is consuming a high protein diet requires more calcium in his or her diet to maintain calcium balance than someone who eats less protein. In situations where dietary calcium intake or absorption is sub-optimal, a high protein diet may further worsen calcium imbalances and increase the risk of osteoporosis." Osteoporosis is a disease that results in the thinning of bones and sometimes fatal fractures. Studies have associated milk consumption with higher rates of osteoporosis. The Harvard Nurse's Study showed that women who consistently drink milk have much higher rates of bone fracture than women who eat very few dairy products or avoid them altogether. As Dr. Willett has said, "There's no solid evidence that merely increasing the amount of milk in your diet will protect you from breaking a hip or wrist or crushing a backbone in later years."

Milk is touted as the ultimate source of calcium, but there are other good sources that do not pose the same health risks, especially to people who are already suffering from serious illness. One cup of milk contains 300 mg of calcium. One cup of cooked collard greens contains 360 mg. One cup of kale contains 210 mg. One cup of cooked bok choy contains 250 mg. Many other green and leafy vegetables are rich sources of calcium, as are many fish. Three and a half ounces of salmon contains 290 mg. The same amount of mackerel contains 300 mg. A tin of sardines contains 480 mg.

In addition, researchers are increasingly concerned about allergens found in milk. In a study published in the *New England Journal of Medicine*, dairy protein was shown to trigger an auto-immune response in certain children, causing immune cells to attack and destroy insulin-producing cells of the pancreas and leading to the onset of juvenile (type-1) diabetes. Population studies throughout the world have consistently shown an association between milk consumption and higher rates of insulin-dependent diabetes. As Dr. Willett has pointed out, about 75 percent of the world's adult population cannot digest lactose, including some 50 million Americans.

People who are lactose intolerant suffer from a variety of digestive disorders when they consume milk, including cramping, diarrhea, nausea, and bloating. Citing the tendency of milk to create constipation, iron deficiency, and allergies in infants, the American Academy of Pediatrics has recommended that parents avoid giving their infants any cow's milk products before the age of one year.

"How dairy foods came to be considered essential despite their high content of fat, saturated fat, and lactose is a topic of considerable historical interest," states Dr. Marion Nestle in her book *Food Politics, How the Food Industry Influences Nutrition and Health.* "As it turns out, nutritionists have collaborated with dairy lobbies to promote the nutritional value of dairy products since the early years of the twentieth century. Recently, however, some scientists have raised doubts about whether dairy foods confer special health benefits. In addition to concerns about lactose intolerance, some question the conventional wisdom that dairy foods protect against osteoporosis or, for that matter, accomplish any public health goals. Others suggest that the hormones, growth factors, and allergenic proteins in dairy foods end up doing more harm than good."

For a healthy person, small doses of unhealthy substances do not pose a significant threat to health. But for someone who is battling a serious disease and already suffering from high inflammation, even small amounts of harmful food can feed the illness. Moreover, threats to human health are found in far greater concentrations in the food supply than in other areas of the environment, such as pollutants in the air, water, or soil, so it makes sense to be vigilant. Each of us has much more control over the harmful substances in food than we do over environmental toxins, which means that changing the quality of your food is the first and most important step you can take to recover good health. On a plant-based diet, you will consume abundant quantities of plant chemicals that can be powerful healing substances against serious diseases.

HEALING NATURALLY

While modern medicine has failed to find answers to so many of the epidemics we face today, the human body already possesses all the abilities needed to reverse major disease and restore health. The truth is that the body has healing powers that scientists, medical doctors, and complementary healers have only begun to understand. In order for the body to utilize its healing forces effectively, however, it needs the right conditions. Among the most important and fundamental conditions needed to restore health is a healing diet. When you begin to understand just how powerful a plant-based diet can be, you will stand back and marvel. That's what scientists are discovering now—that plant foods work in harmony with the body's own healing forces to conquer illness and restore health.

Dr. James Carter and his colleagues at the Tulane School of Public Health found that people with pancreatic cancer who followed a macrobiotic diet lived substantially longer than those who were treated with standard medical care, according to a study published in the *Journal of the American College of Nutrition.* Dr. Carter followed pancreatic cancer patients for one year and found that 54.2 percent of those who had adopted the plant-based diet were still alive one year after diagnosis, while only 10 percent of those who had undergone standard medical care had survived.

A twelve-member panel of scientists at the National Cancer Institute (NCI), a branch of the National Institutes of Health, studied the remarkable case histories of six people who overcame end-stage cancer after adopting a plant-based, macrobiotic diet. These six people had been meticulously documented by medical doctors throughout their recovery periods. All six had been diagnosed with end-stage cancer. All six had adopted a macrobiotic diet and lifestyle after all conventional treatment had failed. All six were still alive and diagnosed as disease-free many years after diagnosis.

Scientist and longtime cancer investigator Dr. Ralph Moss was a member of the NCI's panel, which interviewed all six former cancer patients and reviewed their medical documentation. After examining the evidence, Moss wrote:

> This session [of the NCI panel] brought forth strong testimony that sometimes the adoption of a macrobiotic diet is followed by the dramatic regression of advanced cancers. A nurse told how, in 1995, she was diagnosed with lung cancer that had spread all over her body. She received no effective conventional therapy, and reluctantly went on the macrobiotic diet. . . . What makes this case so extraordinary is that her progress was monitored weekly by a sympathetic physician colleague. The shrinkage, and finally the disappearance, of her tumors was documented millimeter by millimeter! She has now been disease-free for over five years.

As you now understand, the modern diet, rich in sugar, fat, and harmful chemicals, places an enormous burden on the human body, disrupting a vast, interdependent network of biochemical processes. Over time, these dietary substances can trigger a disease process that, depending on your genetic predispositions, ultimately manifests as one or another life-threatening illness. For some, it's a form of cancer; for others, heart disease; for still others, diabetes. Many illnesses that appear to be separate on the surface can actually arise from the same underlying source: a diet that creates chaos within the biochemistry of the human body.

If you are already ill, adopting a plant-based diet may seem like shutting the barn door after the horse has fled, but in the case of your health, a plant-based diet is, in fact, exactly what you need to get the horse back in the barn—meaning, it offers you a clear and scientifically valid approach to recovering your health. Today's most widespread health problems depend on certain biochemical conditions to thrive. Change these conditions and these health problems may improve or, in many cases, disappear entirely. You can cut off the lifeblood of these illnesses by bringing the three factors previously discussed—insulin levels, inflammation, and weight—under control.

A diet composed chiefly of vegetables, beans, cooked whole grains, fruit, nuts, and an assortment of vegetable-based soups and condiments can bring insulin, inflammation, and weight back into healthy ranges. The nutrients and phytochemicals found in plant food can also boost immune function and promote healing. Moreover, many plant-derived chemicals can even change the way genes function. Certain plant substances can cause genes to issue new commands to cells, restoring proper cellular function and allowing diseased cells to commit programmed cell death.

The fact is that an overwhelming abundance of research shows that a diet rich in plant food can relieve people of serious, even life-threatening diseases. Science is learning that a plant-based diet can serve as an adjunct form of therapy for many people who are already ill and searching for powerful ways to heal themselves.

Getting Well

Studies have shown that many people with type 2 diabetes who adopt a plant-based diet, lose weight, and exercise regularly are able to free themselves from the disease and all diabetic medication. Researchers who studied the Pritikin diet and exercise program found that 70 percent of type 2 diabetics who exercised regularly and followed the plant-based Pritikin diet became free of all diabetic symptoms and the need for medication.

A study done by UCLA scientists and published in *Obesity Reviews* showed that men with prostate cancer may improve their chances of

Fiber—The Secret Weapon

Remarkably, plant foods offer protection against cancer not only due to their effects on insulin levels and inflammation, but also thanks to their high fiber content. High-fiber diets help reduce high estrogen levels in the body, which have been linked to cancer. Fiber binds with excess hormones, cholesterol, fat, and other harmful substances, and aids in their elimination through the feces. In fact, vegetarian women eliminate two to three times more estrogen in their feces than do non-vegetarians, according to a study published in the *New England Journal of Medicine*. Fiber's ability to lower estrogen levels in the blood is truly astounding. Plant-based, high-fiber, low-fat diets have been shown to reduce estrogen levels by as much as 40 percent. For women with hormone-sensitive cancers, a significant drop in estrogen levels can mean the difference between life and death.

survival by adopting an insulin-lowering, low-fat diet. Researcher Dr. James Barnard and his colleagues found that men with prostate cancer who followed a low-fat diet rich in whole grains and vegetables and exercised regularly experienced a dramatic drop in insulin levels. At the same time, these men produced more of a particular substance that binds with insulin and helps eliminate it from the body.

One of the reasons a plant-based diet can be effective against cancer may be because it can restore apoptosis, or programmed cell death, in relation to cancer cells. Dr. James Barnard and his co-workers at UCLA discovered exactly this phenomenon in men on a low-fat, plant-based diet and exercise program. The key factor to restore apoptosis, Dr. Barnard found, was returning insulin to healthy levels. Once this happened, programmed cell death was restored and cancerous cells began to die. Cancer cells can become increasingly resistant to medical treatment, so scientists have long been searching for ways to induce apoptosis. Dr. Barnard's study, along with other research, suggests that a plant-based diet coupled with exercise may create an internal environment that is highly antagonistic to cancer.

Preventing Inflammation

Vegetables, fruits, and whole grains fight inflammation in many different ways. One way is by inhibiting a particular enzyme known as cyclooxygenase

2, or COX-2, which produces inflammatory prostaglandins and cytokines. While these inflammatory substances are essential to the body's ability to heal itself and fight infections, an overabundance of them leads to harmful chronic inflammation. Many plant compounds, especially substances called polyphenols (found in vegetables, fruits, tea, and red wine), as well as omega-3 fatty acids (commonly found in flax seeds, some nuts, and coldwater fish such as white fish, salmon, and tuna), can help prevent chronic inflammation by impeding COX-2 and thus discouraging the process.

Plants also fight existing inflammation and its most destructive forces: free radicals, or highly reactive oxygen molecules. Among the most important plant constituents to do this, of course, are antioxidants. Antioxidants reduce and sometimes even stop oxidation, including oxidation of LDL cholesterol, which means they help prevent atherosclerosis. In a highly inflamed, free radical-rich environment, cancer flourishes, in part because free radicals cause ongoing DNA mutation and the continued production of cancer cells. In relation to this fact, researchers have found that antioxidants boost the number and aggressiveness of virtually all immune cells, including natural killer cells, among the most important weapons the immune system has to fight cancer.

Scientists have also discovered that when the tissues contain reserves of antioxidants—a kind of nutrient bank account—immune cells are more aggressive and effective against all forms of illness. Cornell University researchers have found that Chinese people who eat their traditional grain and vegetable diets have the highest blood levels of antioxidants and the lowest cancer rates. They discovered that the antioxidants contained in the diet have a particularly strong effect on natural killer cells and their ability to destroy cancer cells and tumors.

It is interesting to note that women with breast cancer who adopt a plant-based diet low in fat seem to enjoy better outcomes and longer life spans than those who do not make such changes. In fact, Dr. James Hebert and his colleagues at the University of Massachusetts reported that the composition of the diet of women with breast cancer can determine whether the disease returns or recurs once it has been pushed into remission. Recurrence plays a pivotal role in survival. Once cancer recurs, it is often extremely difficult, if not impossible, to force it back into remission. Dr. Hebert and his colleagues found that high-fat foods, including dairy products, were associated with shorter survival among women with breast cancer, while the consumption of plant foods and antioxidants were associated with longer life. Premenopausal women with breast cancer who regularly ate butter, margarine, and lard had a 67-percent greater chance of cancer recurrence than those who avoided these foods.

The antioxidants that we hear most about are vitamins C, E, and beta carotene, the vegetable source of vitamin A. But there are many more, such as vitamin B_6, glutathione, L-cysteine, and several minerals, including selenium, zinc, copper, and manganese. Moreover, many plant chemicals known as phytochemicals act as antioxidants, which means that with every vegetable, piece of fruit, or bowl of grain you eat, you get hundreds—sometimes thousands—of antioxidants. Phytochemicals, in fact, form one of the most exciting subjects in nutrition science. Found only in plants, phytochemicals have myriad functions in the body, including boosting the immune system and fighting diseases such as cancer and heart disease. The following are the most common phytochemicals and some of their health-enhancing effects.

- **Flavonoids.** These substances suppress tumor growth, prevent blood clots, reduce inflammation, and induce apoptosis. They are abundant in apples, celery, cherries, cranberries, kale, onions, black and green teas, red wine, parsley, soybeans, tomatoes, and thyme.

- **Indole-3-carbinol.** This compound is found in cruciferous vegetables, such as bok choy, broccoli, Brussels sprouts, cauliflower, cabbage, collard greens, kale, mustard greens, rutabaga, sauerkraut, and turnips. It can convert cancer-causing estrogens into their more benign forms and thereby help prevent breast cancer. It is also a powerful weapon against prostate cancer. In one study, Dr. Alan Kristal and his colleagues rigorously examined the eating habits of 1,230 men in the Seattle-area between the ages of forty and sixty-four. Overall vegetable consumption provided strong protection against prostate cancer, but cruciferous vegetables had the strongest effects. According to Dr. Kristal, "At any given level of total vegetable consumption, as the percent of cruciferous vegetables increased, the prostate cancer risk decreased."

- **Isoflavones.** These compounds are among the most celebrated phytochemicals. They act as mild estrogens and as such are known as phytoestrogens. In addition to being antioxidants, they block tumor formation, and starve tumors for blood and oxygen. They also prevent bone loss, lower blood cholesterol, and reduce enzymes that stimulate breast cancer. Foods rich in phytoestrogens include soy products, whole grains, berries, fruit, vegetables, and flax seed.

- **Polyphenols.** According to cancer researcher Dr. Michael Wargovich, plant chemicals such as polyphenols are often many times more powerful antioxidants than are simple vitamins such as C and E. Not only do polyphenols act as antioxidants, but they also induce programmed cell death in cancer cells. Polyphenols are found in abundance in strawberries, blackberries, flax seeds, black and green teas, apples, hazelnuts, and whole grains.

- **Saponins.** These compounds are found in whole grains and soy products. They neutralize enzymes in the intestines that cause colon cancer.

- **Sterols.** These are chemicals found mostly in vegetables. They lower blood cholesterol levels.

- **Sulforaphane.** This compound is found in broccoli, broccoli sprouts, Brussels sprouts, cauliflower, cabbage, and other crucifer vegetables. It possesses remarkable anti-inflammatory and anti-cancer properties. Sulforaphane has been shown to kill cancer stem cells, the very root and source from which cancer cells spring. It also stimulates cells to produce an enzyme that protects and restores healthy DNA. Sulforaphane induces cells to differentiate, but can also turn off genes that cause cancer cells to replicate endlessly.

It is important to note that animal foods do not provide important antioxidants such as beta carotene, vitamin C, or phytochemicals. Scientists advise us to eat at least five servings of whole grains, vegetables, and fruits per day to get adequate antioxidants. People who eat fewer than five servings of antioxidant-rich foods each day experience twice the risk of developing cancer than those who get those five servings, says long-time researcher Dr. Bruce Ames, professor of biochemistry and molecular biology at the University of California, Berkeley. One study published in *Nutrition and Cancer* showed that women with breast cancer who took vitamin C and E supplements experienced fewer recurrences and lived longer than women who did not take these antioxidant vitamins.

Of course, a plant-based diet's ability to inhibit inflammation also combats heart disease. The ongoing Nurse's Health Study being conducted by Harvard University has found that women who ate five or more servings of carrots per week had 68-percent fewer strokes than those who ate carrots only once a month. Moreover, research also suggests that women who eat antioxidant-rich foods suffer significantly fewer heart attacks than those

---

Magic Beans

Among the most celebrated of the isoflavones is genistein, which is found primarily in beans, especially soybeans and soybean products. Genistein is especially abundant in traditional Japanese soybean products such as miso, a fermented soybean paste used in soups and stews; shoyu, naturally aged and fermented soy sauce; tamari, the liquid drawn from aged and fermented miso; tempeh, whole soybeans aged, fermented, and made into a patty; edamame, boiled or steamed whole soybeans; and natto, whole, fermented soybeans, used as a condiment on grain or noodle dishes.

Numerous studies have shown that genistein blocks blood vessels from attaching to tumors, preventing them from getting the oxygen and nutrition necessary to survive. This ability, known as anti-angiogenesis, is but one of many cancer-fighting properties of genistein, which also acts as an antioxidant and fights inflammation.

Scientists now believe that the abundance of isoflavones, including genistein, in the blood of women living in Asia may be one reason why these women do not encounter the rates of breast cancer seen in the West, and why women on an Asian diet also have much better rates of survival from breast cancer than do Western women. In relation to males, studies suggest that genistein may prevent dormant prostate cancer from shifting to its malignant phase.

---

who do not. But the adoption of a plant-based diet doesn't just prevent heart disease, it can also reverse it.

Dr. Dean Ornish and his colleagues showed reversal of atherosclerotic plaque in the coronary arteries of heart patients who followed a vegan diet. Numerous follow-up studies have repeated this same finding, including those done by Dr. Caldwell Esselstyn of the renowned Cleveland Clinic Medical Center. Research undertaken by Dr. Richard Fleming also displayed a reversal of atherosclerosis in patients who also followed a low-fat, plant-based diet. Dr. Fleming's study compared the effects two different diets—a plant-based diet low in fat and a high-protein diet—on blood flow to the heart. After one year, the people on the plant-based diet experienced reversals of plaque in their coronary arteries, while those on the high-protein diet experienced progressions of their heart diseases and diminished blood flow to their hearts.

It is clear that a plant-rich diet low in fat and protein combined with regular exercise can, and in many people does, reverse heart disease. For many people, it may also restore normal blood pressure and eliminate the need for blood pressure medication.

Controlling Weight

Excess weight is not only associated with higher rates of illness, but it's also a big factor in determining whether or not a seriously ill person survives. Researchers at the University of Massachusetts Medical School interviewed 149 women with breast cancer to learn their dietary practices and other lifestyle habits. The interviews took place around the time of their diagnoses, after which the scientists followed the women for at least five years. The study, published in the medical journal *Breast Cancer Treatment* reported that those who ate more calories experienced higher rates of recurrence. For every 1,000 additional calories consumed, there was an 84-percent increase in the risk of recurrence. The researchers found that among those women who had consumed more calories, most of those calories had come from fat. Just eating an additional 100 calories per day above the number needed to maintain current weight increased the risk of recurrence by 5 percent. Weight control is an essential part of the healing process.

A plant-based diet is inherently low in calories, which makes losing weight far easier on a diet composed of unprocessed grains, fresh vegetables, beans, and fruit. These foods are also rich in water and fiber, which fill you up without increasing weight. Indeed, people can eat until they are full and still lose excess weight. This fact was demonstrated in a study published in the *Archives of Internal Medicine*, which showed that people on a high-carbohydrate, low-fat diet could eat as much food as they wanted and still lose one pound a week. The diet was made up primarily of cooked whole grains, vegetables, and fruit. The subjects did not exercise and still lost weight.

According to Dr. Alice H. Lichtenstein, professor of nutrition at Tufts University, "It's not excess carbs that translate into body weight, it's excess calories—no matter where they come from." Many scientists are now pointing out that Americans have been duped into believing that all carbs cause weight gain. In fact, the only carbs strongly associated with weight gain are the processed kind (e.g., pastries, bagels, bread, and refined sugar), which are extremely high in calories and cause elevations in insulin.

Complex carbohydrates, which are found in whole grains, fresh vegetables, beans, and fruit, actually lead to weight loss, even when you eat till you are full.

Altering Gene Expression

If there is anything that reveals the power of plant foods to heal, it is the recent discovery that vegetables and fruits alter gene expression in favor of health. In a great many cases, plant foods alter the very genes that play a direct role in the causation and reversal of cancer, heart disease, and other serious illnesses.

At the University of Montreal, Dr. Parviz Ghadirian and his team of researchers have been studying women with the BRCA-1 and -2 genes, which have been linked to increased risk of breast cancer. Up to 80 percent of women who carry these genes eventually develop breast cancer, and as a consequence, many women with these genes elect to have a preventive double mastectomy. In the course of his research, Dr. Ghardirian discovered that a minority of women with the cancer-causing genes did not develop cancer. Upon further study, he found that the women who ate the most vegetables and fruit avoided the illness. He analyzed the women's habits even further and found that those women who ate as much as twenty-seven servings of different vegetables and fruits each week experienced a 73-percent reduction in breast cancer risk. It seemed as though something in the fruits and vegetables was turning off the BRCA-1 and -2 genes.

Research on the human genome has begun to provide answers as to why some women with the BRCA-1 and -2 genes develop cancer while others do not. Scientists have discovered an extraordinary array of chemical compounds that wrap themselves around DNA and instruct genes on what to do—in essence, turning a gene or gene sequence either on or off. These chemical compounds are known as the epigenome. The epigenome acts as a kind of maestro for your DNA, directing and organizing your genetic information to create your unique genetic symphony. According to researchers, your epigenome can be altered by your behavior, particularly by what you eat.

"We can no longer argue whether genes or environment has a greater impact on our health and development, because both are inextricably linked," said Dr. Randy Jirtle, a genetics researcher at Duke University. "Each nutrient, each interaction, each experience can manifest itself through biochemical changes that ultimately dictate gene expression. . . ." Indeed, the more scientists investigate the mysteries of our genes, the more they discover the importance of specific nutrients—and overall diet—as keys to the optimal workings of our genetic inheritances.

At Georgetown University, Dr. Xiantao Wang and his colleagues discovered that compounds in broccoli and other cruciferous vegetables such as cauliflower, watercress, and collard greens target and destroy a specific mutated gene known as mutant p53. The p53 gene is a tumor suppressor, but when it mutates it loses this ability and allows cancer to thrive. But broccoli and other cruciferous vegetables contain substances that work directly on p53. Research has shown that certain compounds in cruciferous vegetables eliminate mutant p53 genes while leaving the functioning ones alone. Remarkably, scientists have also seen ample evidence to suggest that compounds in cruciferous vegetables have the ability to restore function to mutant p53 genes.

Other plant foods have been found to have profound effects on the genome. Soybeans and soybean products such as miso, tempeh, tofu, and natto (a savory, fermented soybean condiment used on cooked grains) have been found to activate 123 genes in the prostate that suppress inflammation and tumor growth and initiate DNA repair. Curcumin, a powerful antioxidant found in turmeric, calms and turns off genes that trigger inflammation. Studies have shown that people who eat regular amounts of curcumin have exceedingly low rates of Alzheimer's disease and urinary cancers.

At the Medical College of Georgia, Dr. Stephen Hsu and his team have found that an antioxidant in green tea called epigallocatechin-3-gallate (EGCG) turns on genes that command cancer cells either to differentiate—meaning to become healthy parts of a specific organ—or to initiate apoptosis, also known as cell death. "In tumors, certain signal pathways become corrupted and stop functioning so that the cells keep growing," said Dr. Hsu's team member Dr. Wargovich. "It's like having the light switch taped in the 'on' position. When that happens in cells, certain functions cause cells to become cancerous. Green tea re-regulates the cell, it reboots the system so to speak, to accept commands to stop growing."

These and many other discoveries reveal that food, especially plant food, can have very powerful effects on our genetics. No form of chemo - therapy or any other type of treatment in the medical arsenal has demonstrated the power to change our genes for the better as plant food has.

Dr. Jeffrey Bland, scientist and best-selling author, points out that there are reasons for the special powers food has on the genome. According to Dr. Bland, "Plant foods are enormously complex. They contain a rich array of minerals, flavonoids, polyphenols, nucleic acids, tecopherols, and tens of thousands of other phytochemicals. As we ate these foods and evolved, we came to depend on these substances in order to regulate gene expression and sustain health. Rather than create messages from the god of war, these foods send very different messages to our genes. They create signaling processes that regulate insulin sensitivity. The regulate cell division and repair. They determine GI function—our ability to absorb nutrients and eliminate waste. They determine the strength and balance of the immune system, and consequently regulate inflammatory responses. All of these functions are harmoniously controlled by eating a diet that is composed of foods that we refer to as minimally processed."

As Dr. Bland has stated, we can see the effects of a plant-based diet on large populations, such as the people who live in the Mediterranean region. "In the Mediterranean diet, animal protein is not the centerpiece, as it is in the American diet. Vegetables, beans, and whole-grain products are the center of the diet. And everything is minimally processed. And if you look at the health of people who follow such a diet, you see that they have lower rates of the common illnesses than we do on a highly processed, meat-centered diet."

WHAT TO DO NOW

A healing diet can be the foundation for your plan to overcome serious illness. Such a diet is rich in colorful vegetables, beans, cooked whole grains, fruit, sea vegetables, and minimally processed natural foods. A plant-based diet will help you achieve the three goals necessary to good health, which are to lower your insulin levels, curb inflammation in your body, and reduce your weight. Your doctor can track each of these measurements over time to monitor your progress. A blood glucose test and a blood insulin test will tell you your blood sugar and insulin readings. A simple blood test known as C-reactive protein (CRP) can give you a baseline inflammation level. Finally, you or your doctor can check your weight against the body mass index (BMI), which is widely available online, to make sure you lose weight and remain at a healthy weight.

In general, a healing diet is composed essentially of the following groups of food:

- At least three servings per day of green and leafy vegetables, such as bok choy, broccoli, Brussels sprouts, cabbage, cauliflower, collard, kale, mustard greens, Chinese cabbage, or watercress.

- At least two servings per day of sweet vegetables, such as rutabaga, turnip, squash, onion, sweet potato, or yam.

- At least two servings per day of root vegetables, such as burdock root, carrot, daikon, dandelion root, ginger root, lotus root, parsnip, red radish, rutabaga, and turnip.

- At least one serving per day of beans, such as aduki beans, black beans, chickpeas, kidney beans, lentils, lima beans, navy beans, or soybeans.

- Two servings or more per day of cooked whole grains, such as amaranth, barley, brown rice, buckwheat, millet, oats, quinoa, or whole wheat.

- A variety of whole-grain pastas.

- Sea vegetables, including Atlantic alaria, nori, dulse, kombu, and kelp.

- A variety of fruit.

- Pickled or fermented plant foods, such as cucumber, ginger, sauerkraut, miso, tamari, shoyu, or numerous other fermented or pickled foods.

- If animal food is desired, eat white fish as your first choice and salmon as your second.

This diet is not only healing but delicious, especially when you learn how to prepare the ingredients in a number of tasty ways. Once you have your diet in place, it will be time to look at other aspects of your life as you seek to promote your healing further. And the next big step will be to start bringing more love into your life.

CREATE A SUPPORTIVE COMMUNITY

Until this point, the healing process has been largely an individual experience, requiring you to concentrate on the actions you alone can take to restore your health. But when you arrive at this step, you will encounter a larger message: You can go no further on your own. You need others to help you now.

If you are coping with a serious illness, the notion that you can get well all by yourself is a dangerous illusion. To borrow a well-worn concept, it takes a village. Those who get well do so, in part, by creating a supportive and life-enhancing community around themselves. The healing path unfolds before you as a growing web of connections to people and new knowledge. As you make these connections and benefit from the support and knowledge you receive, you will realize that the essence of the healing journey is expanding love—the love you give to others and the love you receive from those closest to you as well as from those you meet along the way.

Like a varied bouquet of flowers, love comes in many forms. One form, of course, is the love that comes from a spouse or partner. Others include the love that comes from family and friends, from healers and teachers, from support groups and social organizations, and from clergy and spiritual leaders. Opening yourself up to the many forms of love and receiving them with gratitude are acts of self-love and, indeed, of self-healing.

At this point, you are being challenged to create a network of healing relationships based on various forms of love. In many cases, you must ask for and accept help, care, and love from many different kinds of helpers, including professional healers and medical workers. You will very likely turn to relatives, friends, and neighbors who can help you with many small but important chores. In some cases, however, your requests for help will be much more personal and intimate.

You will be asked to heal conflicts in your most important relationships. Forgiveness of others, being forgiven, and forgiveness of self are central challenges on the healing journey, and such work is especially important now. A pivotal place has now been reached, a place at which you realize that in order to heal your body you must act from your heart.

LOVE, BIOLOGY, AND HEALING

What is love? No definition can fully capture the transformative power of this sacred force. But in order for us to have some working understanding of love, allow me to offer my own definition, which is this: Love is the giving of energy that nourishes and supports life. Love is the act of perceiving in your heart what someone might need at any particular moment and then giving that life-enhancing gift freely, without conditions, and even with joy.

Love flows through many mediums. It flows through a person's touch. It is in a person's caring eyes or happy smile. It's in music that soothes, relaxes, or inspires you. It's in healing words, compassionate attention, insight, forgiveness, and celebration. Love is in every expression of true gratitude. It's in dance, art, and sport. It is in every expression of joy. Among love's most salient characteristics are its freedom from fear and its power to dispel it. As St. John wrote almost two thousand years ago in 1 John 4:18, "There is no fear in love, but perfect love casts out fear, because fear involves punishment and the one who fears is not perfected in love." We may begin to understand love's power to heal once we understand love's amazing effects on human biology. These effects become even more impressive when compared to those of fear. This contrast is best illustrated by the autonomic nervous system (ANS), which regulates all involuntary functions of the human body, including the cardiovascular system, gastrointestinal tract, urinary function, hormonal function, sexual response, metabolism, bodily fluid production, dilation and contraction of pupils, smooth muscle function, and many other biological activities.

The ANS is divided into two branches—the sympathetic and parasympathetic—which respond to environmental stimuli in opposite ways. The sympathetic branch is activated whenever you experience stress or fear. It triggers the fight-or-flight response throughout the body, elevating stress levels further. It releases stress hormones, including the catecholamines, which include epinephrine (also known as adrenaline), norepinephrine, and dopamine. It speeds up heart rate and respiration, elevates blood pressure, and contracts muscles throughout the body, (including the heart muscle). It raises blood glucose, insulin, and blood lipids, impairing circulation and contributing to heart disease. It slows saliva production, digestion, and motility, and causes bowels to contract. It increases oxidation and, when activated chronically, speeds aging and weakens the kidneys, adrenal glands, heart, bones, and immune system. It also causes weight gain, loss of muscle mass, and impaired memory function.

Love and related emotional states such as compassion, kindness, and deep relaxation stimulate the parasympathetic nervous system, which causes a relaxation of muscles, more restful sleep, and slower heart rate and respiration. It reduces stress on heart, lowers blood pressure, and increases feelings of safety and well-being. It increases production of saliva and digestive liquids, enhancing digestion, motility, and intestinal function. It also boosts production of the anti-aging hormone DHEA and stimulates antioxidation within cells, which also slows aging and disease processes. Finally, it enhances immune response and leads to faster healing times.

Obviously, both branches of the autonomic nervous system are essential to life, as are the emotional states associated with them. The challenge lies in establishing a healthy balance, or to be more specific, limiting fear to short-term episodes—for example, the instant you cross a busy street and realize a big truck is hurtling toward you. Short-term episodes of fear are not the problem. It's sustained stress that can be extremely toxic and potentially deadly. Hans Selye, the pioneer stress researcher, found that prolonged stress can destroy the kidneys and heart. An abundance of scientific evidence has shown that chronic stress can lead to depression, a weakened immune system, serious illnesses, and death.

If you want good health, you need love and all its related state of consciousness, including compassion, kindness, and understanding. Love boosts all the biochemical functions that strengthen the immune system and support the restoration of good health. We are social beings, dependent upon each other for this invisible force that binds us to each other—a force we associate with emotional states, but, as it turns out, one that is just as essential to physical health.

LOVE, COMMUNITY, AND HEALTH

The first major study to demonstrate a connection between social bonds, health, and mortality rates was the Alameda County study, which examined the relationship between lifestyle and health. In 1965, researchers began to track the health and mortality rates of 10,000 randomly selected residents of Alameda County, California. While initial findings showed a link between longer lifespan and five key practices—which included avoiding smoking, exercising regularly, maintaining a healthy body weight, sleeping seven to eight hours a night, and limited consumption of alcoholic beverages—later analyses took social networks into account. The scientists found that those people who regularly attended church or civic organizations, were married, or had close friendships lived longer and were far healthier than those who did not have a strong social network or relationship.

The Alameda County study results have been consistently replicated in many other studies throughout the world. The more isolated a person grows, the more prone he or she becomes to dying prematurely. Some studies have shown that isolated populations have three- to-five times the mortality rates as those who feel connected within their communities. Remarkably, some research has found that isolation is as strong a predictor of health and mortality as blood pressure, cholesterol level, or cigarette smoking.

Supportive and loving relationships can be such a strong promoter of health that they can sometimes counteract harmful habits. In the 1960s, scientists Steward Wolf and John G. Bruhn began studying the people of Roseto, Pennsylvania, who, despite high-fat diets and sedentary lifestyles, experienced much lower rates of senile dementia and mortality from heart disease and stroke than neighboring communities. At least on the surface, it appeared that the Roseto residents were doing everything wrong, yet somehow they were healthier than their neighbors.

After closer scrutiny, the researchers concluded that the good health enjoyed by the Roseto residents flowed from a single factor: their close-knit community. The people of Roseto were primarily Italian immigrants, whom sociologists often refer to as "urban villagers"—so named because they retained their communal traditions even after they moved to new urban settings. The Italian Roseto residents tended to marry other Italians within their community. In fact, it was common for their households to be made up of three generations of family members. They were religious people who were highly supportive of each other, participating in both church and social organizations. Rosetoans were particularly responsive to anyone in their community who had fallen on hard times or were faced with a crisis. They provided love, care, and feelings of security, all of which contributed to their overall good health and low mortality rates.

These conclusions were reinforced when, by the end of the twentieth century, many Rosetoans began to turn away from their traditional ways of living, only to subsequently experience a sharp increase in their disease and death rates. As Wolf and Bruhn observe in their book, *The Power of Clan: The Influence of Relationships on Heart Disease,* many Rosetoans gradually became more affluent, materialistic, and less socially cohesive. Its members became enamored by expensive cars and bought bigger houses that were outside of Roseto. Their church attendance dropped dramatically and many married outside their community. Soon, their rates of heart disease and other illnesses were as high as or higher than those of the average Americans.

LOVE IS A HEALER AND A TEACHER

Love has a way of getting past our defenses and touching our hearts. Once you let love inside, it strengthens your entire being, including your healing forces. You become stronger somehow, more resilient, and better able to heal. In a study done at Duke University, researcher Dr. Redford Williams and his colleagues studied people who had had heart attacks and found a pronounced difference in health outcomes for those who had a loving spouse or partner, versus those who were forced to try to recuperate alone. "What we found was that those patients with neither a spouse nor a friend were three times more likely to die than those involved in a caring relationship," said Dr. Williams.

Well-known immunologists Dr. Janice Kiecolt-Glaser and Dr. Ronald Glaser have conducted numerous studies on how the quality of relationships affects the immune system. In one study, the researchers compared the immune systems of married women, each of whom was given a questionnaire to determine the quality of her marriage. In general, the immune systems of married women were healthier than those of unmarried women, but it was the quality of the relationship that had the greatest impact on health. Those women who said they had loving and supportive husbands also had stronger immune systems than those who said their marriages were difficult and unsupportive.

The Glasers found similar results in men. Unhappily married men had weaker immune systems than happily married men. Even more telling, the men who were separated had the weakest immune responses of all.

In the absence of love, our fears grow like a deepening night until they engulf us in the darkness of isolation, self-doubt, and even self-hatred. Love, like the dawn, can send the shadows fleeing. Love illuminates and magnifies the best in us. It alters our perception of what's possible to achieve in this life. Indeed, it gives us a glimpse of our heroic nature, our ideal selves, allowing us to be more creative, more powerful, and less afraid.

We can see new possibilities and perform feats that our lesser selves would not attempt or even believe possible. Our heroic nature is the part of us that gives life meaning. And, needless to say, it is also the part that can heal us of disease.

Only when you love can you come fully into your power to transform yourself and others. Your love must manifest first as love for yourself, which must include practical acts of self-love. Love must guide you in all your health habits, such as your dietary choices, your exercise regimen, your need for rest, your need for gentle touch, your need to be heard and understood, and your need to be alone. Your love of self will allow you to recognize toxic relationships and to gently eliminate them from your life, while encouraging you to spend time with people who love you and support your healing.

Part of love's healing effects must certainly come from the fact that love unifies, creates bridges, and brings together that which has been separated. If it were not for the unifying force of love, conflicts would have no way to reconcile, which means people in conflict would have no means to reconcile, forgive, and find peace. Love makes life possible. And once it exists in a relationship or situation, it opens up possibilities for growth, creativity, and the very best in each of us.

Love allows us to glimpse the lofty worlds that live inside us all. But we cannot fully occupy these worlds until we learn to love others. Until we love consistently, we are trapped in a childlike relationship with those around us, secretly waiting for others to give us the love we need so we can feel strong and secure enough to be our best selves. Waiting for others to love us first makes us into powerless victims. We shrink from life and settle into our lesser selves, the part of us that is fearful and angry for not getting the love we need.

Love that is real is, in fact, an action. The love you give to others makes you supportive, understanding, and compassionate. In this way, your love inspires those around you and, in the process, makes you the creative force in your relationships. The more you love, the more you set the tone in your relationships. Your ability to love transforms you from victim to creative catalyst. As you support others and make them aware of their own best selves, you naturally shift into your own heroic nature, or higher self, which is the realm from which miracles may flow.

Love shines a light on the good and the beautiful in people. In doing so, it encourages these qualities to grow. Those who love express more praise than criticism, more tenderness than discipline, more understanding than intolerance. The person who genuinely sees the good in others and then promotes that good is giving nourishing love and enhancing the lives of those he or she encounters.

There are many ways to promote the good in another. It can be done with simple statements of appreciation—"You are so good at that," or "What you did took tremendous courage," or "I am so grateful you have been there for me"—or through simple acts such as finding ways to lift a loved one's burden, however small, so that his or her life is a little less difficult. When expressed out of genuine love and appreciation, your words and actions can transform both their recipient and your relationship with that person. Together you become two people who are not on constant alert for criticism from the other. As your love for each other deepens, you become two people free of defense, free to put down your armor. You are no longer confined to your own small self and your own intense self-doubt, which arises when your mistakes are emphasized.

Every great coach has used love to bring out the best in an athlete. Among the preeminent practitioners of this approach was Angelo Dundee, the trainer for the great boxer Muhammad Ali. Dundee realized early on that Ali responded badly to all forms of criticism. So, whenever he wanted Ali to throw a punch in a particular way, he wouldn't instruct him negatively, but rather he would find a way to instruct through praise. "I love the way you throw that jab just like this, champ," Dundee would tell Ali, miming what he wanted done. Ali would get the message and follow suit. Dundee saw the greatness in Ali and helped to bring it forth with relentless love.

Authentic love in the form of praise or belief in a person's inherent talents or goodness awakens the life force in its recipient. It brings forth powers that were latent and asleep but in the light of love suddenly surge into being. Through authentic love, we are suddenly more than our ordinary selves. We can accomplish feats we previously believed were impossible. This is the nature of love: It elevates the life force and makes the best in us possible.

OVERCOMING THE BARRIERS TO LOVE

Expressing love isn't always easy. Human history is defined more by fear and trauma than by love. Fear of attack causes us to erect barriers against each other, and against the giving and receiving of love. Those barriers are hard to take down, even when we want to restore love to a particular relationship. When this happens, there is only one way back: through forgiveness.

Certain relationships are crucial to your psychological health and well-being. Only you can determine which of your relationships fall into that category. Your essential relationships may be with your wife or husband, a life partner or long-time friend, your children, or your mother or father or both. Whatever the nature of the relationships, one thing is certain: Forgiveness has been essential to maintaining the free flow of love between you and the people you care about. In fact, you've probably had to forgive these people not once but many times, just as they may have had to forgive you. Forgiveness is love's best friend. Without it, love cannot endure.

We have all witnessed countless examples of the living hell that is created when two people in an essential relationship don't embrace forgiveness. In many cases, they are relegated to lifeless conversation (which is often hurtful in its silences), passive-aggressive sniping, or outright verbal war, even as the two people remain inextricably linked and committed to staying together. Sadly, many people in such relationships secretly hope that the other person will soften and express remorse for what has happened between them. Each mistakenly believes that something said in anger will somehow soften the other's heart. Of course, such hopes are illusions. Pain only causes more pain.

If you find yourself in this type of situation, your heroic nature may begin to whisper a single question to you over and over again: How can I forgive and get back to love? Below are six steps that can help you forgive and restore love in an essential relationship. While these steps may be used to promote forgiveness in any relationship, I am suggesting that they be used only in essential relationships, at least for now. Sometimes we complicate the subject of forgiveness by including non-essential relationships in our discussion. You may ask, "Do I have to forgive the person who attacked me, or stole my wallet, or took away my job?" Only you can say whether you need to forgive that person. If the anger and hatred are eating away at you and thereby serving as impediments to your health, then perhaps the answer is yes. But at this moment, you may not be ready to forgive a non-essential person for the hurt he or she may have caused you.

A much more important relationship may require forgiveness in order for you to restore the love between the two of you. Forgiveness may represent a much bigger step in your healing process, especially in the creation of a greater sense of peace in your life. Here are six steps that can help you forgive someone you love and restore the flow of love between the two of you.

Give Up the Need to Be Right

Conflicts are sustained when each partner insists that he or she is right and the other is wrong. Being right is a powerful and seductive illusion. Within it lies a relentless yearning for victory, a yearning that will not let you rest until you are vindicated. Unfortunately, many people take this yearning to their graves still unsatisfied. Meanwhile, the campaign to prove you are right has the effect of molding you into a frustrated, hardened, and embittered person who secretly longs to be loved but is deprived of love in part by the stubborn defense of your position.

If there is a single lesson to be learned in all essential relationships, it is that there are always two truths present in every disagreement. Even when one or both of you are unable to fully express your feelings, your respective truths are nonetheless equally real. You have your own personal needs, experiences, and perspective; so, too, does your friend or family member. Until each truth is understood and expressed, you cannot know what is motivating your actions or those of your partner, nor can you come to a true and lasting peace.

In a relationship that is driven by the need to be right, real listening is impossible. Instead, you find yourself furiously thinking about what you will say as soon as your partner takes a breath. Every fiber of your being is dedicated to proving the other person wrong and annihilating that person's truth in the process. Only when each of you recognizes that you have an incomplete understanding of the other's truth—and allows the other's truth to be expressed—may understanding, compassion, and love be restored. The best approach, therefore, is to give up being right. Instead, try to understand the needs and motivations of both yourself and your partner. Know that we all yearn to be understood, validated, and loved.

Accept Responsibility

In all essential relationships, neither party is free of error. Find your own mistakes, however buried inside they may be, and admit them to yourself. Once you have reflected upon them, confess them to the person with whom you are in conflict. Acknowledge that your error hurt the person you love. Promise this person that you will do everything in your power to avoid making these mistakes again. Apologize and ask for forgiveness.

Your honesty, courage, and vulnerability will change your relationship with the person you love. More important, it will also change your rela-tionship with yourself. We often insist on being right to avoid facing the underlying awareness of our own mistakes. When we confess our mistakes, something inside us relaxes and celebrates our reconnection to truth and the Divine.

In the mid-1990s, I wrote a long piece about a medical doctor who volunteered much of his time in the hospice ward of his local hospital. One day, I followed him on his rounds and spoke to the people who were dying, and to whom the physician administered palliative care. Every person I interviewed put forward the same message: Love, forgiveness, and honesty were the most important lessons in life, they told me. Those who expressed their love honestly and directly, who forgave others and were forgiven, were also at peace at the end of their lives.

Later, the doctor told me of a former patient who had a wife and four children, all of whom he had abused with his violent temper. By the time he arrived at the hospice ward, he was ninety-three years old and had only weeks to live. The proximity of death made him realize how sorry he was for the way he had treated his family. Deeply humbled, he begged his wife and children to forgive him for his abusive behavior. He told each of them how much he loved them. "I was so hard on my children that I ruined my family," the doctor recalled the man saying. "My anger came from my fear. I always believed that if I didn't do things just right, my life would be ruined. What could happen, I didn't know. I had too much pride. I was arrogant. I wanted everyone to reflect well on me. If they didn't behave just as I wanted . . . "—he made a gesture with his hand, indicating that he would hit them.

Miraculously, the man's full confession and humble plea satisfied a deep need in his wife and children and elicited their love. "I remember how that family huddled around him at the end," the doctor recalled. "His approaching death drew them closer to each other, and the love they all felt for each other was a beautiful thing. Were all their wounds healed? No; of course not. But when someone important to you acknowledges that he or she has hurt you and then begs for your forgiveness, you are changed in a positive way. Your wounds begin to heal. You experience some form of justice and a kind of closure. You can love yourself more, and you can even start the process that leads to forgiveness of the one who hurt you. That is very healing."

That is love. Remember Gandhi's statement: "Where there is love, there is life." And for those who sought the courage to face themselves, he offered the following: "God is truth." When we admit our own mistakes, we experience greater wholeness and reconnection with our hearts and all that is right in the universe. And in the process, we are redeemed.

As a short word of warning, I would like to add that most of us have been so well trained in self-defense that we sometimes use confession as a tool for manipulating our loved ones into making their own confessions. We start out confessing our own mistakes and then end up accusing our loved ones of failing to reciprocate. This is not the point of this step. There is only one goal: to honestly state how you have contributed to the conflict with the person you love, with no other expectations. Only by making such a confession can you enjoy its rewards. In any case, your partner will know whether or not you are sincere. Any sentiment that is less than sincere will backfire and reinforce your conflict.

Share Your Gratitude

All your essential relationships have great meaning, if only because these people have filled such important roles in your life. Conflict with these people—your spouse or partner, children, friends, parents—tears at the soul and changes the quality of your life. Consider how much of a contribution your loved one has made to your life. Experience your gratitude for this contribution, and express how important it is to you.

Not long ago, a couple came to see me for health advice and support for their marriage. I asked each person to consider why he or she needed the other, and what each did to enrich the other's life. The man spoke first and listed the many reasons he needed his wife, and what she gave to him. When he finished, she was in tears. "It's so good to hear that," she said. "I didn't know you felt all of that. I didn't even know that you noticed." He was equally moved when she expressed all the reasons she needed him. Each was fulfilling a role in the other's life that was unique and irreplaceable.

There is only so much time in this life, the body teaches us. When reflected upon, this fact should serve as a reminder of what is truly most important.

Find a Healthy Outlet for Your Emotions

Practicing forgiveness does not mean you have to abandon your feelings and truths. You may still have many emotions—anger, fear, disappointment—that you need to acknowledge and explore. Seek the help of a compassionate therapist who can lead you deeper into your memories and feelings and thus help you understand and love yourself. Your doctor, friends, or clergy member may be able to recommend such a person. As well, many massage therapists, especially those who do therapeutic massage, Reiki, or healing touch, encourage their clients to express the deeply held emotions that often arise during their healing sessions.

If you choose to write about your pain in order to reach a state of forgiveness, express your anger, frustration, or feelings of betrayal or abandonment, but don't stop there. Don't linger too long in blame of others or of yourself. Too much time spent dwelling on your critical feelings will serve only to reinjure you. Instead, write with the intention of moving past these hard, critical thoughts to the tender states of sadness, compassion, and forgiveness. As much as possible, consider the gentleness, innocence, and vulnerability that still live inside you and others, no matter what has occurred. These are the healing forces that live inside all of us and contribute to our recoveries.

See the Other as Happy, Fulfilled, and Healed

To be truly free, you must release yourself from feelings of revenge, retribution, and anger that you may hold for the person who injured you. This is especially true for the person whose love is essential to your life. This work can be accomplished by envisioning the loved one with whom you have been in conflict as happy, fulfilled, and healed of any injuries or pain he or she may have suffered—injuries and pain that ultimately may have caused this person to hurt you, as well. See your loved one as whole and joyful. Imagine him or her free of the binding constraints of anger, fear, and disappointment. See him or her as loved by many, but especially by someone special.

As you project this image outward, your affirmation becomes a powerful prayer that is broadcast as a life-affirming image, one that will transform your inner world. And as research on prayer and quantum science has shown, your prayer also has the power to affect the life of the one for whom you pray and hope will heal. By holding the image of this person in your heart and mind—an image of him or her as healthy, happy, and fulfilled— you are, in fact, freeing yourself from any negative feelings that may have been binding the two of you to each other, thus contributing to both forgiveness and freedom. This is the act of forgiveness, transforming your inner world and that of the person for whom you pray.

As you do this work, you will discover how liberating it is and how much it transforms your inner life, making you much happier, more positive, and emotionally lighter. You will find that as you forgive another, you will feel forgiven for the mistakes or actions you still hold against yourself, and for which others may hold against you. True forgiveness goes in both directions—you forgive another and find that you are forgiven as well.

GETTING THE LOVING CARE YOU NEED

In order to do all this work, you will need support, especially in the form of love. One of the best ways to get this support is by regularly receiving energy and love from a practitioner of healing touch. Touch is an essential form of love that, ideally, should be experienced many times each day. Studies have shown that infants and young children who are deprived of touch often have weaker immune, endocrine, and digestive systems. They are also more likely to experience heightened emotional and mental stress, adverse hormonal conditions, antisocial behavior, and a greater tendency to violence.

When a group of such children underwent regular therapeutic massage, they experienced increased levels of serotonin, the brain neurotransmitter that elevates feelings of well-being, confidence, and relaxation. As serotonin rises, levels of dopamine—the neurotransmitter that promotes aggressiveness and stress—decrease. Studies of adults have shown similar results—that therapeutic massage increases brain levels of serotonin, promotes feelings of well-being, improves sleep, and encourages states of deep relaxation. By touching the body with love and care, the practitioner can soothe the mind and relieve the body of long-held distress.

In a great many cases, that old distress has been held in the body since childhood. During times of verbal or physical violence, a child's first reaction is to recoil in fear and shock. With repeated attacks, this reaction becomes habitual and locks in the physical and emotional pain—even the memories of these events—in the fibers of the body. If there is intense and repeated physical abuse, the shock, fear, anger, and sadness held in the body become even more acute.

The physical recoil manifests in the body as a contraction of muscles and other tissues, restricting range of motion and preventing the circulation of blood, oxygen, immune cells, and lymph. Like a clenched fist, these contracted tissues can hold waste products in the form of carbon dioxide, metabolic byproducts, and stagnant lymph and tissue fluid for decades, making these areas of the body perfect breeding grounds for disease. A trained and talented healer will know how to touch these affected areas so that the muscles learn to relax, restoring the flow of blood, oxygen, immune cells, and lymph to affected areas.

This same state of contraction and spasm exists on a cellular level, especially as a consequence of inflammation, which often causes tissues to swell and circulation to be blocked and stagnant. Even more, adept healers are able to direct electromagnetic energy to weakened or wounded parts of the body.

Dr. Elmer Green, a physicist formerly at the Menninger Foundation, used highly sensitive equipment to test the quantity of electricity that healers could produce and transmit. Dr. Green connected electroencephalograph amplifiers to the copper walls and ceiling of his laboratory so that he could measure the electrical output produced by ordinary people as well as by adept healers. He found that ordinary people at rest—meaning standing still, with normal heart rate and respiration—produced between 10 and 15 millivolts (a millivolt is one-thousandth of a volt). Dr. Green's cohort of healers was capable of producing 190 volts per individual in single sessions. Obviously, 190 volts is far above the 120 volts available in an ordinary American wall socket, and more than 100,000 times greater than normal human electromagnetic output.

Dr. Robert Becker, an orthopedic surgeon and professor of medicine at State University of New York, Syracuse, studied the changes in electrical impulses produced by the body during the process of healing. Dr. Becker found that whenever the body engages in healing—either wound healing or eradicating an infection—the body increases the flow of electromagnetic energy to the affected area. Dr. Becker showed that an affected part of the body sends a "stimulating signal" to the brain, indicating the presence of a disorder—either an injury or infection. The brain responds by increasing the electrical charge flowing to that part of the body, thus stimulating cells to initiate healing. As the body repairs itself, the intensity of the signal decreases, which diminishes the flow of electrical current to the wound. Eventually, the disorder is healed and no stimulating signal is sent at all.

One of the complementary healing systems that Becker studied extensively was acupuncture, which is among the primary healing tools of traditional Chinese medicine. The Chinese maintain that the life force, or qi, flows through the body in 12 distinct channels, or meridians. Along these pathways of energy are acupuncture points, which are said to act as generators of energy when stimulated, either by the shallow insertion of a needle at the point's precise location on the skin, or by applying finger pressure or heat. By stimulating the acupuncture point, the healer increases the flow of energy to the organ associated with that meridian. This increase in energy provides the basis for the restoration of health.

In his book *Cross Currents: The Perils of Electropollution, the Promise of Electromedicine*, Dr. Becker states, "We found that about 25 percent of the acupuncture points on the human forearm did exist, in that they had specific, reproducible, and significant electrical parameters and could be found in all subjects tested. Next, we looked at the meridians that seemed to connect these points. We found that these meridians had the electrical characteristics of transmission lines, while nonmeridan skin did not. We concluded that the acupuncture system is really there, and that it most likely operates electrically."

According to Dr. Becker, numerous healing tools can boost electrical charges throughout the system and thus promote healing. In addition to acupuncture, Dr. Becker found that a healing diet, herbs, homeopathy, massage, visualization, and placebo all generate increases in electrical flow at infected or injured sites within the body. Acupuncture, in fact, has been the subject of considerable scientific research. The World Health Organization maintains that acupuncture is effective in the treatment of more than sixty disorders.

The works of both Drs. Becker and Green, along with other research, provide a possible explanation for how practitioners of therapeutic touch are able to promote healing by increasing the flow of electrical energy to an effected part of the body. Penn State's Milton S. Hershey Medical Center reports that therapeutic touch can be effective in a wide array of disorders, including chronic pain, allergies, sleep apnea, fibromyalgia, lupus, bronchitis, and addiction. Researchers have found that therapeutic touch speeds wound healing. Some studies suggest it may promote healing through healthy cell growth. Therapeutic touch also has been shown to relieve headaches, and reduce pain, and improve function in those who suffer from arthritis.

In her book *The Touch of Healing*, Alice Burmeister describes the gentle but powerful art of Jin Shin Jyutsu, an ancient healing technique that uses gentle touch to balance the body's energy pathways. She reports many remarkable case histories of people who used Jin Shin Jyutsu to recover from serious illness. One of those people was Amy Tandy. Suffering from severe kidney disease for more than ten years, Amy had gradually lost all but 21 percent of her kidney function. Her doctors insisted that if it fell to 20 percent, she would require immediate kidney dialysis and a kidney transplant. She was forty-nine years old. One day, after seeing her physician, she sat in her car in a state of shock. What could she do? Suddenly, some inner strength welled up inside of her. She was not going to have dialysis or a transplant, she decided. She was going to find her own answers.

Amy had recently begun seeing a bodywork therapist who practiced Jin Shin Jyutsu. Each Jin Shin Jyutsu session left Amy feeling noticeably better—more relaxed, energetic, and optimistic. Following the hard news from her doctor, Amy began to undergo these treatments three times a week. She also did a Jin Shin Jyutsu self-help routine—a form of self-massage—every day. She gave herself over to Jin Shin Jyutsu completely, and in a matter of two months found that her kidneys were becoming stronger. When her kidney function crept up to 30 percent, her doctor was amazed. "If you get up to 40 percent," he told her, "I'll learn this Jin Shin Jyutsu." After a year, her kidney function reached 43 percent. Her physician told her that there was no longer any need to discuss dialysis or transplant. Unfortunately, all her doctor would say after Amy's dramatic health improvement was that he could not explain her recovery.

Picture yourself, full of stress, lying on a healer's table. Someone with a gentle healing touch applies his or her hands to your tightened shoulders, painful back, swollen rib cage, cramped legs, and tortured feet. Slowly, these parts of your body start to relax and release tension as your body learns to trust the compassionate love that flows through your therapist's hands. Your breathing gets slower, deeper, and more rhythmic; your muscles surrender their tension and release more energy into your body; and your long-held misalignments start to come back into balance. The biological impact of such changes is enormous.

Healing massage, therapeutic touch, acupressure, and acupuncture can help relieve many of the physical and psychological conditions that support your illness. Healing touch will comfort you, alleviate stress and tension in your body, and provide tremendous comfort as you do the important work of healing. It will promote the forces of healing that are rising in you right now. It will show you that you are not alone in your struggle—there are people walking with you who are committed to your recovery.

WHAT TO DO NOW

You probably cannot simply go out and form your own version of Roseto, Pennsylvania. What can do, however, is create a network of healers who support you with their own special skills, abilities, and compassion. By working with a wide array of medical and complementary healers, you can form your own personal community of healers and enjoy many of the same health-enhancing effects as those experienced by the Roseto residents.

When choosing a complementary or medical practitioner, the guiding light should be both expertise and skill in a particular field of knowledge, and his or her ability to communicate ideas with compassion, understanding, and wisdom. To find the right practitioner, ask your medical doctor, hospital nurses, and clergy members for referrals. There are online services that either rate practitioners or provide comments from people who have experienced the work of specific healers. Once you sit down with a healer, ask if he or she has worked with people who suffered from the same condition as your own or a condition like it, and what the experience was like for both client and practitioner.

Find a Practitioner of Therapeutic Touch

Therapeutic touch is one of the world's oldest forms of healing and is practiced in churches, synagogues, and temples across the country and around the world. Many practitioners who are associated with a church or temple will perform healing touch for a nominal fee, or will do it for free. In addition, many nurses are professionally trained practitioners of therapeutic touch. Your doctor may know several good nurse-practitioners. If not, call your local hospital and ask for a referral.

There are many forms of therapeutic massage and healing touch. Among the most widely practiced are acupressure, shiatsu, chiropractic, craniosacral therapy, deep-tissue massage, therapeutic massage, bioenergetics, Reiki, Jin Shin Jyutsu, and Swedish massage. Be sure to choose a practitioner who has been trained by a reputable massage or chiropractic school. (See Resources on page 217.) There are many excellent schools for various forms of massage and therapeutic touch throughout the country. Most of these schools need volunteer patients on which students may practice in order to develop their skills. In many cases, these sessions are provided free of charge or for minimal fees.

Find a Dietary Counselor

Health professionals who specialize in various diet and lifestyle programs can be found all over the country and around the world. These practitioners can coach you in your dietary choices and teach you how to prepare healing foods. Among the plant-based programs with numerous available counselors include the macrobiotic diet and lifestyle, the Pritikin Program, the McDougall Program, and programs associated with Dr. T. Colin Campbell or Dr. Caldwell Esselstyn. (See Resources on page 217.)

Join a Healing Community

Communities associated with specific healing practices—especially dietary and lifestyle programs—may be found all over the country. Such communities can provide enormous support and practical information about healing. Often, they also offer a wide variety of services, including cooking classes, potlucks, and social support. You are very likely to find people who are facing or have faced similar health challenges to your own.

Many churches, synagogues, and temples provide healing services associated with specific religious traditions. Ask a clergy member if your church or temple offers any such services.

Find a Mental Health Counselor, Therapist, or Life Coach

Many towns and communities offer low-cost psychological counseling programs. Believe it or not, many state departments of mental health offer free psychological counseling to anyone who cannot afford such counseling. These services can be found online, and a good place to start searching would be the online yellow pages (www.yellowpages.com) under "Social and Human Services."

Identify Someone You Would Like to Forgive

One of the most powerful initial steps you can take in clearing your heart and opening the way in your search for healing is to restore a relationship through forgiveness and being forgiven. For all the reasons already spoken, when you bring healing forgiveness to your loved ones you will experience greater healing yourself.

Join a Support Group

Most cities and local communities provide support groups for virtually all of the most common health challenges. People in these groups may exchange vital information and personal experiences with medical and complementary care. Local people can provide referrals for doctors, nurses, and complementary practitioners of every type. Members will not only share information but also compassionate support, simply because many of the people in such groups understand what you are going through as few others can. Support groups are among the most important sources of guidance, care, and practical information available. Learn from other people's experiences

Thankfully, the Internet has made it easier than ever before to find support groups and services for every demographic group. You can use any search engine to find support groups for specific health issues. You can also use facebook (www.facebook.com) to search for and become a member of support groups of all types. Finally, you may also find various types of charities in connection with your illness, which may either help you directly or refer you to other helpful organizations. As you develop your network of healers—your loving community—your program will begin to take a clear shape.

COMMIT TO HEALING

ommitment is a lion lunging upon its prey. It is a new mother getting up at 3 AM to attend to the needs of her newborn child. It is a performer stepping onstage, ready to give all he or she has to the anticipating audience. Commitment is you focused on the details of your daily actions—choosing healing meals over greasy, processed, sugary foods; getting up a little earlier to take a walk or do your exercises; and spending a little time in prayer. Commitment is you stopping all that you are doing to give loving attention to someone who needs you at this very moment. Commitment is you living in integrity with your purpose. It is the process by which you are transformed physically, mentally, emotionally, and spiritually—the method by which you are forged anew to become your healthier, stronger, better self.

When you commit to reaching a goal, your actions take on greater power. They are suddenly imbued with the invisible healing power of spirit. With spirit comes love, and suddenly, the miraculous is possible. Making a deep and sincere commitment to healing is a vital step in your recovery process.

The foundation of commitment is made up of three qualities. The first is the ability to know your own heart—which is to say, to know what is true and right for you. Your heart is a channel of love and life energy. In fact, ancient Chinese sages once taught that all living things are imbued with a life force, or qi, that animates the human body and, when strong enough, heals the body of any disorder, illness, or wound. When your heart is in alignment with a course of action, your body is infused with energy and feelings of inspiration, or enthusiasm, or balance. Conversely, when your heart rejects a particular idea or approach, you may experience your body contracting, rearing up, and withdrawing your life force, all because you intuitively know a particular action is wrong for you. These emotional and physical reactions can offer practical help when faced with challenging decisions. Listening to your heart and knowing deeply that a particular course is right for you are the ways to true commitment.

The second quality is the courage to follow your heart. Once you know what is right for you, take the time to sit with this knowledge and be present with this deep intuitive feeling of what is right. Let it become part of you. In a short while, you will be filled with the courage to walk your path in harmony with your heart.

The third quality is focus—the ability to concentrate, or bring your awareness to your actions. In fact, focus is what directs your life force to your actions and your goal. For example, a person who concentrates his or her life force on a particular work of art may produce something far more beautiful, powerful, and true than a person whose energies are scattered across many different activities.

Commitment is the basis for consistency of action, and thus a source of great power. Consistency can make you surprisingly strong, like the relentless wind that reshapes a rocky cliff, or the constant flow of water that can wear away an entire coastline. This is an especially important idea when using alternative or complementary medicine, both of which are directed more toward eliminating the supporting aspects of an illness and building up the body's own healing mechanisms. These approaches require time and consistent action to deliver their full healing power.

HOW TO STRENGTHEN YOUR COMMITMENT

One activity above all others can strengthen your ability to commit to a healing program: regular physical exercise. Exercise, like no other behavior, strengthens your will power and your capacity to maintain a healing routine. It also makes all your healing behaviors stronger. You do not need to adopt any sort of complicated or particularly demanding exercise regimen in order to experience the vast benefits of regular exercise. You can start out simply by taking a daily walk. You can also adopt some other form of gentle exercise, such as yoga, or stretching, or a gentle martial art, such as tai chi chuan or qi gong. Of course, before starting any exercise regimen, consult with your physician to make sure it is safe to do so. It is also a good idea to undergo regular physical examinations so that you can monitor your progress and ensure that you are not hurting yourself.

With continued and consistent exercise, your stress levels will fall. Your feelings of optimism will rise. You will start to believe in possibilities you could not even see before you began exercising. Remarkably, other health-promoting activities will also become more effective and powerful, especially your ability to adhere to a plant-based, healing diet. In fact, scientists have found that exercise is the single greatest factor when it comes to predicting whether or not a person will remain on a healing diet.

The effects of regular exercise on dietary patterns have been an intriguing subject for researchers, especially the effects of exercise on cravings for certain types of foods. This was the focus of a study done by Dr. Peter Wood and his colleagues at Stanford University, who studied a group of middle-aged men who jogged every day for two years. The researchers gave the runners no nutritional advice, but closely monitored their dietary choices throughout the two-year period. The men who exercised also experienced an increase in their appetites. This was to be expected, since they had raised their caloric outputs. It was notable that the men changed their diets to include more unprocessed plant foods, which are rich in complex carbohydrates. Of course, as the body's primary source of energy, carbohydrates were being burned off quickly through exercise. But what was truly remarkable in Dr. Wood's study was that the health-promoting effects of exercise seemed to extend to the food choices the runners made. The men were attracted not to sugar or processed food but instead to complex carbs from pulpy vegetables, legumes, and whole grains.

Eating complex carbs from unprocessed food lowers insulin levels, which, as previously mentioned, can lead to an array of incalculable health benefits. Exercise also elevates HDL cholesterol (the so-called "good cholesterol" that protects against heart attack and stroke), lowers blood pressure, and strengthens the heart muscle and improves its efficiency (meaning the heart pumps more blood per beat). In addition, exercise reduces the stickiness between blood platelets, thus improving circulation and lowering the risk of blood clots.

Moderate exercise significantly strengthens the body's fight against cancer by increasing both the number and aggressiveness of all major classes of immune cells. With regular moderate exercise, the immune system is far more aggressive and effective against disease-causing agents, including cancer cells and tumors.

Finally, exercise strengthens bones, increases muscle mass, and elevates mood significantly by increasing brain levels of endorphins, the body's natural opium-like compounds. Some studies have shown that regular moderate exercise can be as effective as medication in the treatment of mild to moderate depression.

Exercise is maintained when one is committed. Indeed, exercise is the visible and living expression of commitment. And in commitment lies the magic of healing, as Ralph Donsky experienced firsthand.

RESOLVE TO SURVIVE:
RALPH DONSKY'S HEALING ODYSSEY

Ralph Donsky was about to go on vacation with his wife and two daughters to Ocean City, New Jersey. As he lifted the last of the family's bikes onto his car's roof rack, Ralph felt a stabbing pain shoot through his back. The pain was so intense that, according to Ralph, it "knocked the air out of [him] and caused [him] to bend over and put [his] head between [his] legs to catch [his] breath." Ralph was relieved when the pain gradually disappeared. Undaunted, he and the family made it to Ocean City and had a pleasant and uneventful vacation.

Three weeks after Ralph got home, the pain returned. It was just as intense as it had been originally, but this time it was no longer confined to his back but also radiated throughout his rib cage. Over the next few days, it got worse. Soon, he couldn't sit for more than fifteen minutes without intense and terrible pain that spread throughout his ribs and down his spine. Alarmed, he went to his family doctor, who could not find anything wrong with him. The physician referred Ralph to an endocrinologist, a specialist in conditions related to hormones. Ralph underwent an exhaustive series of tests. When the test results came back, there was only one conclusion: Ralph had Cushing's disease.

In Cushing's disease, tumors or excessive growth in the pituitary gland set off a chemical chain reaction ending in the excessive production of the stress hormone cortisol. At such high levels, cortisol prevents bones from absorbing calcium, which was why Ralph's bones were deteriorating. The weight of his body was too much for his bones to carry. It wasn't long before Ralph couldn't stand or lift even a light object without breaking a bone. He was forced to lie in bed in a slightly elevated position in order to prevent the weight of his body from placing too much pressure on his spine.

The brain tumor thought to be causing Ralph's case of Cushing's disease would have to be removed, his doctors said. By removing the tumor, the doctors hoped to stop the hormonal cascade that had led to his bone loss. Unfortunately, MRIs could find no evidence of a tumor. His doctors decided that the only course of action was to remove Ralph's entire pituitary gland, under the suspicion that the tumor was there but too small to detect. His pituitary was removed, but after thorough analysis, no tumor was found. Meanwhile, the disorder continued to stimulate Ralph's body to produce high levels of cortisol and his bones continued to crumble.

Ralph was placed on high doses of morphine, which dulled his mind as well as his pain. The drug drained him of his energy and distorted his perception. Every one of his movements seemed to occur in slow motion. It took him two hours to eat a meal. At times, he felt as if he were floating inside a giant pool.

A month after the surgery, Ralph suffered a massive heart attack. He was rushed to the University of Connecticut Health Center, where he fell into a coma for five days. When Ralph emerged from the coma, he found himself in the critical care unit, attached to a multitude of wires and tubes. Suddenly, the memory of months of pain, broken bones, and crumbling vertebrae came rushing back. He sunk into his pillow and felt despair engulf him. *How was he going to face the future?* he wondered.

A few days later, Ralph's doctor explained that Ralph's adrenal glands would have to be removed. Unable to find the tumor itself, the theory was that by taking out his adrenal glands, Ralph's body would stop making cortisol and his bones would gradually be able to absorb more calcium. Without the surgery, Ralph's bones would continue to deteriorate, his doctor said. By then, Ralph had already lost six inches of height and was now standing five feet four inches tall. If this process didn't stop, he would soon be dead.

The surgery could not be done immediately—his heart had not recovered sufficiently to withstand the stresses associated with the operation. When Ralph returned home again, he was shocked by the severe curvature of his spine. "I looked like the hunchback of Notre Dame," he said. "I worried about how I was going to face the world in this disfigured state." Far worse, however, was the intense back pain that he suffered. "I was in continuous pain for eighteen months," Ralph said. "I couldn't ride in a car for more than five minutes because the position it put my back in was too much for me to bear." He was still given daily doses of morphine, which left him feeling as if he were living inside a dream—a dream rife with pain and fear. The fear and the pain opened up a dark portal inside of him and allowed all his demons to emerge.

"I was afraid of going to sleep at night," Ralph recalled, "thinking that I would not wake up in the morning. I was also afraid of the dark. I correlated darkness with my life coming to an end. The pain, the drugs, the surgery on my pituitary gland, and my heart attack had all combined to wreak havoc on my mental state."

All of this terrified and exhausted his wife and children. "Sometimes my family couldn't bear it anymore," Ralph recalled. "I was depressed and obsessing. It was too much for my family to deal with." Four months after Ralph awakened from his coma, surgeons removed both his adrenal glands, and his bones finally started to heal. This process was facilitated by daily injections of calcitonin, a drug that promotes the uptake of calcium by bones. So began his long and arduous journey back to health.

Ralph's heart attack had occurred because of his Cushing's disease, his cardiologist told him. The illness had caused a blood clot to form in his coronary artery, and this clot had blocked blood flow to the left side of his heart, causing that part of the heart to die.

"How can I prevent that from happening again?" Ralph asked.

The only way to prevent any further danger, his cardiologist said, was to keep his arteries free of cholesterol plaque. The arteries needed to be clean. The only way to do that was by following a strict diet and getting exercise.

Already familiar with the Pritikin program (his father- and mother-in-law had adopted it to treat their own health problems), Ralph began eating a diet composed strictly of whole grains, vegetables, beans, and fruit. He emphasized the green vegetables such as broccoli and collard greens because of their calcium contents. He also took a calcium supplement. In no time, Ralph became an adept cook, learning how to prepare his meals so that they were delicious, satisfying, and therapeutic all at once.

As for exercise, he knew he had to start slowly. Any exertion terrified him. He was afraid of breaking a bone or having a sudden heart attack. His father had given him a stationary bicycle, which he started riding for five minutes a day at five miles an hour. This small effort exhausted him. "Don't give up," he kept telling himself. "It's not going to get better overnight. You've got to commit to the long haul if you are going to make it all the way back," he said to himself.

Ralph told his cardiologist that he wanted to get to the point where he could ride for an hour before breakfast every morning. "You can do it," his doctor told him. "But you have to go very slowly and carefully." The doctor told him to extend the duration of his workout by five minutes every two weeks. The important thing, said his doctor, was consistency. "If you maintain consistency," the cardiologist said, "you'll be able to reach your goal." Soon Ralph hit upon a single phrase that would become his mantra: Resolve to survive. He repeated this mantra to himself even when he was in severe pain. The phrase embodied his complete commitment to his healing approach, and to life itself.

Slowly, his strength improved. Ralph looked around for an additional form of exercise and found an aquatic workout class in a local health club. The pool was kept at 92°F. Its warmth made his body feel relaxed and capable of exercising when he entered the water. The exercises, done with barbells, consisted of rowing motions and swirling patterns executed under the resistance of the water. The resistance of the water was ten times that of the air. The bike strengthened his legs; the water aerobics fortified his arms and upper body.

"The aquatic workout was an incredible confidence builder," Ralph recalled. "I went twice a week, every week, for three years. When I started, I could barely move the plastic barbells through the water. With time, I became one of the strongest members of the class, almost stronger than the instructor. I remember my incredible determination and resolve. Once I started gaining some muscle back, there was no stopping me."

Meanwhile, Ralph continued to adhere strictly to his plant-based diet. He permitted himself a single serving of chicken or fish once a month. "I made up this diet, based on the Pritikin program," Ralph said. "Pritikin allows a small amount of fat in the form of low-fat animal products, but I wanted to eat a stricter diet that was even lower in fat," said Ralph. "I would not back down on this."

Having established a morning workout routine, Ralph added tennis twice a week, and basketball once a week. The results were nothing short of astounding. Six months after he started this routine of bicycle riding and aerobic workouts, he was riding his bicycle for a full hour at a minimum of twenty miles per hour. Sometimes he would increase his speed and get up to thirty-five miles per hour. Although still small of frame, Ralph had created extensive muscle development in his arms, shoulders, back, abdomen, and legs. In some respects, he was in the best physical condition of his life. He had transformed himself.

Fifteen months after he was diagnosed with Cushing's, Ralph finally returned to work. He wore a back brace and still suffered some pain, but it was significantly diminished. Although he was recovering physically, he was still struggling with his fears. Before long, Ralph fell into a deep depression.

"There is no isolating your mental health from your physical health," Ralph would write years later. "Your brain, which drives all of your bodily functions, also is the recipient of your pain and anxiety. After fighting a severe physical illness, my mental health had suffered as a victim."

Ralph knew it was time for him to heal his mind. He plunged himself into therapy. He also saw a variety of healers. Just as he had done with his physical illness, Ralph addressed his mental and emotional issues with commitment and resolve. It took him one year (just over two years since being diagnosed with Cushing's disease) to make a full recovery—physically, mentally, and emotionally. He no longer experienced any pain. He was free of the back brace. And all his tests—including his tests for heart disease—showed that he was in excellent health. Remarkably, his body was no longer producing abnormally high levels of cortisol. On the contrary, his hormone levels were now normal. Somehow, Ralph's medical and personal self-help methods had combined to restore his health.

"I'm back to being a normal guy," he said. "No, I'm even better. I'm stronger than I ever was. I can't believe it, on half a heart."

His doctors shook their heads in amazement. Ralph's cardiologist said, "Ralph, if you had not taken care of yourself the way you have, you would not be standing here in front of me." Another doctor told him, "Ralph, you are alive today because of who you are as a person. You are responsible for where you are today." His psychological health was just as good. All symptoms of anxiety and depression were gone.

"Life is full of surprises," Ralph said. "Sometimes the greatest adversity can bring out the best in a person, and the worst. But if you resolve to survive, good things can happen, even when it seems like everything is falling apart."

HEART RATE VARIABILITY

The metaphorical heart is the place from which true commitment springs—from its courage, honesty, and healing power. But recently, scientists discovered a mysterious role in healing that is played by the literal heart. It is a function referred to as heart rate variability (HRV).

Heart rate variability refers to the intervals of time that occur between heartbeats. It wasn't too long ago that the heart's beat-to-beat rhythm, known as heart rate, was considered a stable activity with little fluctuation. But this idea has changed in recent decades. Now scientists recognize that the heart's rhythm is highly complex, with tiny but highly significant fluctuations between every beat. These fluctuations, scientists have discovered, provide great insight into understanding a person's health status, as well as his or her vulnerability to premature death. Heart rate variability is now seen as a crucial piece of information to have when maintaining or regaining health.

For many decades, scientists who studied the heart believed that a stable heart rate—meaning a consistent number of beats per minute, with the same time intervals between beats—indicated good health. But then researchers began to see a correlation between stable heart rates and greater incidences of illness and premature death. People with low heart rate variability—meaning a consistent heartbeat rhythm and the same intervals between beats—had higher rates of illness and death than others within their age groups. On the other hand, people with greater heart rate variability—meaning a varied number of beats per minute and fluctuating intervals between beats—had more robust health and were less prone to premature death. These findings ran across virtually all illnesses and age groups. Infants with low heart rate variability were more susceptible to sudden infant death syndrome (SIDS) than infants with higher HRV. Adults with low HRV were more prone to all major illnesses, including heart disease, cancer, and diabetes, than adults with relatively higher HRV.

With further study, scientists found that low HRV was associated with prolonged exposure to the sympathetic nervous system. As previously explained, the sympathetic nervous system is responsible for increased stress, higher rates of oxidation, elevated heart rate, elevated blood pressure, and a weakened immune system. Those who experienced ongoing stress were more likely to have low HRV and therefore were more prone to illness and early death. Conversely, high heart rate variability has been shown to be associated with extended periods of parasympathetic nervous system activity, and thus slows heart rate, lowers blood pressure, boosts immune function, and promotes healing.

Thankfully, low HRV does not have to be permanent. Indeed, scientists have shown that HRV can be modified through exercise to promote good health. One of the early proponents of this idea was Dr. Irving Dardik, who realized that long distance runners got sick and died at higher rates than sprinters. From these facts he gained remarkable insight. Dr. Dardik showed that all exercise is essentially a wave, with the rise of the wave associated with energy expenditure—the actual period of exercise—and the decline of the wave with rest and recovery—the "cool down" phase.

During exercise, the body burns energy and thus increases stress, oxidation, and the breakdown of cells and tissues. During the recovery phase, the body gathers energy and experiences an increase in antioxidation, rest, and recovery off energy. Antioxidation, gathering energy, and rest are all essential aspects of the body's healing process.

Dr. Dardik showed that when people exercise for long periods—as long-distance runners do—and do not follow these long periods of stress with equally long recovery phases, the body's healing ability becomes weaker. When consistent long-term exercise is followed by only short or cursory recovery phases, the body spends far too much time in the sympathetic nervous system. As a consequence, it can lose its ability to recover altogether. At that point, it becomes susceptible to illness, without the strength to recover. On the other hand, short periods of exercise followed by committed periods of rest and recovery actually strengthen the body's ability to heal.

Dr. Dardik and other researchers in the field presented a new approach to exercise. No more of the "no pain, no gain" approach. Instead, their findings recommended short periods of relatively high energy output followed by equal periods of recovery time. Dr. Dardik pointed to tennis as an ideal example. During a tennis match, players exercise intensely for short periods—less than a minute on many occasions, rarely more than two minutes. This intense exercise is followed by a period of rest, in which both players gather energy while one player waits for the other to serve the ball.

This specific way to exercise focuses not just on the stress and energy expenditure of physical activity but also on the recovery, or healing, phase. This approach can easily be applied to any form of exercise in which you would like to engage. Take walking, for example. Start your walk at a pace that you feel is in harmony with your energy levels. As you walk, feel and listen to your body and its energy levels. When you're ready, speed up a bit and maintain this pace for a short duration—one to five minutes. Make a

Awakening

A sincere commitment to healing can awaken the spiritual forces that lie deep within you. These spiritual forces may be the real source of your recovery—even if your recovery is attributed to a particular medicine, surgery, or alternative approach. Scientists know very well that without a commitment to health, or to life itself, the immune system mysteriously weakens, and for some even shuts down.

As Ralph Donsky's story reveals (see page 88), healing isn't just a physical experience but also a psychological experience. Endeavors to heal physically often lead to the darkness of doubt, fear, trauma, and harmful beliefs—all of which were lurking within you long before any illness manifested. As you commit to your health, the journey may force you to confront the darker aspects of your heart and soul, which require healing, too.

habit of walking in these patterns, meaning periods of greater intensity and faster speeds followed by periods of strolling, energy recovery, and healing. Do not push yourself beyond your limits. Instead, just get your heart rate up a bit. You should be able to talk and exercise at the same time. If you cannot talk and exercise, you are overexerting yourself and not doing the kind of exercise that will increase your HRV.

Walk for thirty minutes or so. Don't push things, especially at the beginning of your training. After you have finished your walk, initiate a cooldown phase in which you stroll slowly, do some very gentle stretching, and feel your entire body come to a place of peace, harmony, and balance.

COMMITMENT LEADS TO THE LIGHT

It's easy to say that we should exercise, eat a more nutritious diet, join a support group, or meditate and pray. If doing these things were as easy as listing them, we all would be a lot healthier. But something inside us stops us from engaging in such healing activities. Indeed, something compels us to engage in behaviors that are self-destructive and even promote self-loathing.

The moment you commit to a healing path is the moment you must learn to overcome any resistance to healing. This resistance can block you from making progress and plunge you into despair and depression. You may feel alone in your struggles, and as a result you may not feel capable of positive action. Immersed in these dark nights of the soul, you may be forced to ask yourself, *What blocks me from doing what I know to be right?* You are in good company when asking yourself this question. In the depths of his own despair, Saint Paul confessed, "For the good that I would, I do not, but the evil which I would not, that I do." Saint Paul was acknowledging his own resistance to engaging in right action and following what he knew to be the right course. His statement reminds us that we often behave in ways that are both self-destructive and hurtful to others, despite knowing what is good and right. Facing your pain, you may wonder, *What can I do to escape this despair?* The first thing you must do is understand the source of your suffering, and then you may act in gentle ways to relieve it.

As Swiss psychiatrist Carl Jung has shown, we are driven by opposite forces: light and darkness, good and evil, altruism and selfishness. These opposites are inescapable. And the more we deny our darker impulses, the stronger they become. Jung maintained that we repress all urges, drives, and behaviors that do not conform to our idealized images of ourselves. They coalesce into a kind of secondary personality that Jung called the "shadow." The shadow contains all the desires and urges that a person would like to keep hidden but sometimes expresses nonetheless, often in secret ways.

Commitment to healing means facing your shadow. In fact, this is a fundamental part of the healing process—bringing those aspects of yourself that you have repressed or denied into the light of love and acceptance. This confrontation with the darkness within each of us can seem like an eclipse of the sun. But like all eclipses, the light is restored by movement. The light is still within you. The power and desire to heal is there. But in order to rally these healing forces, you must express some of the darkness— and in the process release some of its related tension—so that the impasse can be overcome. It is important to realize that even this painful moment is part of the healing process. Indeed, many great and inspiring insights can be experienced by understanding the conflict and pain that wants to be brought into the light of your awareness.

Some time ago, I interviewed a woman who had a longstanding weight problem. For years, this woman believed that this problem stemmed from her lack of discipline, for which she berated herself regularly. When she reached her mid-thirties, she felt compelled to deal with early experiences of sexual abuse. She entered therapy and joined a support group. Eventually, she discovered that her weight issues were the result of her complicated feelings about men. On the one hand, she feared relationships with men so intensely that she was using her weight as a way to keep men at a distance. On the other hand, she also yearned for a healthy, loving relationship with a man. This yearning led to intense internal conflict, anxiety, sadness, and physical tension—all of which she relieved with food. This emotional eating, of course, helped keep her overweight. As her therapy progressed, she became more conscious of her fears and her desires for a relationship. She began to develop compassion for herself and for her own needs. She learned that, as an adult, she had the power to determine how a relationship developed, and how close or intimate anyone could be with her. This was a power she did not have as a child, but one that she would have to learn to use in order to find satisfaction and balance in her life.

This awakening gave her the confidence to start dating, and to search for a fulfilling relationship, which she eventually found. As she became more fulfilled, she did not have to turn to food to satisfy needs for love and tenderness, and she went on to lose almost all of her excess weight as a result. In my interview with her, she told me, "You know, I didn't realize it, but I wasn't just keeping men out of my life—I was keeping a lot of good things away. I was spending my life protecting myself from the very things I needed, and using food to compensate for my empty life. I was starving and I didn't know it."

Serious illness is often the consequence of a lifetime of imbalances that arise when we repress needs and impulses that have long been buried in the shadows. These buried elements of our natures attempt to reintegrate and reunite into our waking lives. They start to push against our conscious minds like water against a dam. The more they do so, the more tension we experience. This tension can manifest as anxiety, fear, anger, or the need to speak our truths and to be loved. It is common for us to turn to food, cigarettes, alcohol, drugs, television, or video games to reduce the tension that arises when repressed needs, long buried, start to surface. Too often, food can be seen not only as a source of nutrition but also as a source of love and self-medication. Ice cream, chocolate, cookies, pastries, potato chips, soda pop, hamburgers, and French fries are known as comfort foods, and the fact that these foods dominate our food supply says a lot about how much suffering exists in society today. There can be no doubt that these foods, when eaten in excess, can lead to life-threatening disease. We can only postpone the pain for so long before it rears its head and takes control of our lives, oftentimes in the form of illness.

The emergence of an illness can become the moment when you open up to your pain and attempt to restore some degree of balance to your life. To do this, you must examine your deeper urges, which long to be expressed, and allow them to emerge from the shadow and into the light of consciousness, acceptance, and love. You can make the shadow conscious by using a very simple process developed by psychologist Dr. James Pennebaker.

Dr. Pennebaker studied the effects of confession or self-expression on the immune systems and psychological health of college students. He found that the people who wrote about their traumatic experiences had dramatically stronger immune responses and made fewer visits to the health clinic than those who did not write. Moreover, Dr. Pennebaker found that the most profound improvements in immune strength occurred in the people who made the fullest confessions, meaning that they confessed feelings and events that they had never before expressed, even to themselves. Many of these people, whom he called "high disclosers," thanked him profusely for giving them the opportunity to tell their stories.

After the study, Dr. Pennebaker theorized that the transformative power was catharsis. He pointed out that inhibition, the mechanism by which we keep the contents of the shadow hidden, even from ourselves, requires a certain amount of psychic and physical energy. As he puts it, inhibition is a demanding form of work, especially when very painful events or memories must be kept secret. Inhibition, Dr. Pennebaker found, is frequently associated with an array of physical symptoms, including a weakening of the immune defenses and elevations in blood pressure, heart rate, breathing, skin temperature, and perspiration levels. These and other symptoms disappear when we no longer have to struggle to keep the contents of the shadow hidden, but instead allow it to emerge and become conscious.

You can use what has become known as the "Pennebaker method" to release parts of your shadow into the light of awareness and compassion. The exercise is simple and cost-free. You simply take at least twenty minutes each day for four days and write about the most traumatic experience of your life. You should write about the same experience over the four-day period. Once you have spent four days examining this one experience, you can do the exercise again, writing about another painful experience you have had.

Dr. Pennebaker found that during the first two days of their writing experience, the study's subjects wrote about negative emotions such as anger, sadness, anxiety, or grief. On the third or fourth day, however, the participants tended to release their negative emotions and experience relief, insight, and resolution of those feelings. This finding suggested to Dr. Pennebaker that the sufferers had managed to integrate the traumatic events into their consciousnesses. The energy that had been devoted to negative emotions was then available to be rerouted and used for improvements in physical and immunological health.

Dr. Pennebaker suggests you adhere to four rules while doing the exercise:

- Write only about the single most upsetting experience, trauma, or shame-filled event of your life.

- Write about this event or experience for at least twenty minutes of each of four consecutive days.

- Don't worry about the grammar, spelling, or structure of the piece.

- Write your deepest thoughts and emotions regarding the experience. Include all the details you remember as well as any insights into the events. Make a full confession of all that you feel, especially your darkest feelings. The more you confess in your diary, the greater the impact the act of writing will have on your psychological and immunological health.

Once you have finished writing, share your work with someone you love, or with a therapist, healer, or religious or spiritual figure. Let this confession be the basis for an enriching treatment.

Dr. Pennebaker found that people who do this exercise begin to see themselves and their experiences in a different way. Indeed, many discover that their former guilt is replaced by compassion for themselves, newfound self-respect, and far greater self-love.

Remember that you do not have to stop using your diary after writing about a single experience. Rather, give yourself some time to integrate the writing exercise and the insights that emerge from it into your conscious mind. Once you are ready, take up pen and paper again and write about other painful experiences, or whatever you are going through at that moment, using the same formula outlined by Dr. Pennebaker: twenty minutes a day for four days.

WHAT TO DO NOW

As you practice your healing program and begin to change, new questions will emerge from within you. You will wonder, *To what am I really committing, and what am I becoming?* You are committing to your survival and to a healing program that you believe can help you recover your health. You are taking good care of yourself. You are forgiving those closest to you and seeking forgiveness. You are practicing greater love for yourself and others. You are evolving as a human being. A new version of you is emerging. Slowly, you are realizing that your commitment is no longer fueled by fear alone. Rather, you are seeing yourself in a new light, a light that reveals the best version of yourself.

At this point, you know that becoming a wiser, more spiritually alive version of yourself must be part of your commitment. To be sure, the need to survive is driving you, but new thoughts have crept into your awareness and have also become part of your motivation. Something altogether good, something that can only be called spiritual or soul-based, has begun to take hold. Another dimension of life has become available to you. Your commitment has led you into the larger world of faith.

You must now search yourself deeply and find the strength within you to commit to your life and a healing regimen that will support your recovery. If you feel it is right, make a declaration to yourself in writing. Turn this commitment into a daily regimen of healing foods and exercise. Exercise in rhythm. Walk, do yoga or stretching, or engage in some form of rhythmic martial art, such as tai chi or chi gong. Exercise in such a way that elevates your heart rate for periods of one to five minutes, depending on your health status and conditioning. Then rest for an equal period of time and allow your heart rate to fall into the normal range. Try to exercise for about thirty minutes, four to six times a week.

Do the Pennebaker method regularly. Over the course of four days, write for at least twenty minutes a day about traumatic or painful experiences, especially memories that may be emerging as you attempt to heal yourself. Also, write about all the negative feelings you may be experiencing. Express your anger in full, but write with the intention of getting past your anger and experiencing compassion for yourself. Use the Pennebaker method to explore and purge painful memories or struggles you may be having with your healing program. In addition, speak to your healers and a counselor or therapist about any struggles you may be having with your healing program, or any experiences of despair, doubt, or depression with which you may be wrestling.

Consider writer William Hutchison Murray's statement of encouragement:

> Until one is committed, there is hesitancy, the chance to draw back, always ineffectiveness. Concerning all acts of initiative and creation, there is one elementary truth the ignorance of which kills countless ideas and splendid plans: that the moment one definitely commits oneself, then Providence moves too. All sorts of things occur to help one that would never otherwise have occurred. A whole stream of events issues from the decision, raising in one's favor all manner of unforeseen incidents, meetings and material assistance which no man could have dreamed would have come his way. I learned a deep respect for one of Goethe's couplets:
>
>> Whatever you can do or dream you can, begin it.
>> Boldness has genius, power and magic in it!

ℬELIEVE IN YOUR ABILITY TO HEAL

"Believe in yourself! Have faith in your abilities! Without a humble but reasonable confidence in your own powers you cannot be successful or happy." So begins Norman Vincent Peale's *The Power of Positive Thinking*, published in 1952. These words, written more than sixty years ago, are as true today as they were when Peale first wrote them. They are relevant not only to success and happiness but also to the restoration of health. In his book *Anatomy of an Illness*, writer and medical investigator Norman Cousins, who developed his own recovery program to heal himself of the crippling illness described in the book, puts the matter succinctly, writing, "Drugs are not always necessary. Belief in recovery always is."

Words like "belief" and "faith" lead us into a mysterious realm where laws and possibilities transcend those of ordinary reality and every day expectations. Your beliefs, subjective as they are, can infuse your healing program with tremendous power. Your faith can change the course of your disease. Native American medicine man Rolling Thunder used to say that even a glass of water can be powerful medicine if the person believes sufficiently in the water.

It's time to ask yourself what you really believe. Do you believe in your healing program as well as your ability to recover? Are you optimistic about your chances?

Optimism is far more under your own control than you might think. You can learn to be more optimistic. Researchers from the University of Pittsburgh Medical School, Yale University, and Pittsburgh Cancer Institute successfully trained people with cancer to be more optimistic and to overcome self-defeating beliefs. Not only did the researchers succeed in causing the participants of the study to have a positive outlook, but they also found that a positive outlook dramatically improved the immune systems of the subjects.

The scientists examined the effects of optimism-training on thirty patients, all of whom suffered from cancers that had an extremely high probability of recurrence. "The course was designed to make them more optimistic about events in their lives," said Dr. Martin Seligman, a psychologist at the University of Pennsylvania and one of the researchers involved in the study. This optimism translated into very real improvements in the strength of their immune systems. As their levels of optimism grew, participants experienced an increase in the number and aggressiveness of their natural killer cells, one of the most important types of immune cell in the body's fight against cancer.

In his book *Learned Optimism,* Dr. Seligman identifies ways in which you can develop and strengthen your optimism. Among the methods he recommends are:

- **Avoiding negative people and situations.** Be discerning with people. Ask yourself if the person you are interacting with offers life-supporting words and behaviors or instead drains you of energy and positive thoughts.

- **Honoring and celebrating your talents, abilities, and strengths.** Everyone is blessed with their own unique gifts and special talents. Identify your gifts and acknowledge how you have utilized your abilities to contribute to your life and the lives of others. It can be a very healing exercise to write about how your efforts, strengths, talents, and character have benefited your family, friends, associates, and profession.

- **Reading inspiring literature.** Articles and books that reveal how people overcame adversity or brought creative solutions to challenging situations can restore your faith in yourself and the power of the human spirit. Many people find that regularly reading sections of any of the great religious texts—the Judeo-Christian Bible, the Bhagavad Gita, the Vedas, the Upanishads, the Koran, or Buddhist sutras—can be especially effective at boosting your faith and elevating your outlook.

- **Learning to shift your perspective.** There is a silver lining in everything. Make an effort to find it on a daily basis. As you do, witness how the discovery of this positive thread affects your body, mind, and spirit. Finding the good in situations and people is a life-affirming act, one that can move you to be more positive about yourself and life.

■ **Using supportive words that promote the positive.** Dr. Seligman points out that the common phrase "Yes, but . . ." is a shift into more pessimistic thinking and expectations. It weakens any positive thoughts that might have been spoken. Become more aware of how you use words to create a picture of the present or the future. As you become more aware of your words, try to turn things toward the positive. Use phrases such as "I can do that," "my dietary approach is helping me," "my exercise program is making me stronger," "I can feel the progress I am making," and "I am grateful for the help I am receiving." Repeating these sentences on a regular basis will make you more optimistic about your future and have a positive effect on your present.

GRATITUDE

One of the most powerful tools for transforming your life is gratitude. At least twice a day, make a conscious effort to experience and express gratitude for whatever positive gifts life has given you thus far. In a state of true gratitude, you can experience deep humility and freedom from anger and resentment. The grateful person accepts and receives love. Being grateful is an inherently loving state of being. The love and support of your spouse or partner, family, friends, or professional healers may be experienced as an ongoing stream of gifts that you receive in your heart and for which you are truly thankful. Whenever you express genuine gratitude, your heart opens, which, in turn, makes you feel less alone and more connected to others.

Offer words of praise and heartfelt gratitude to those you love, to every helper along the way, and to a power greater than yourself, which brought supportive people, information, and healers into your life. Experience the changes that gratitude causes in your physical body, mind, and emotional and spiritual life. Gratitude can have an almost instantaneously positive effect on you. In moments of gratitude, you are restored to the here and now. Gratitude grounds you in the present. At the same time, it opens your mind to what is truly positive, nourishing, and beautiful in the moment. Giving thanks brings you into an intimate connection with your life and awakens you to the presence of the Divine. And even as you experience gratitude for what you are receiving, in some mysterious way you become a magnet for even more love and more support.

As we have seen, optimism strengthens your immune system, which means optimism makes you stronger in body, mind, and heart. And just as an optimistic state of mind can help you transform your health, improvements in your health can boost your sense of optimism. As long as your immune system has not been irrevocably weakened, your body still possesses awesome healing powers that are capable of overcoming disease. But for your healing program and your body to be sufficiently powerful to restore health, you must believe in them. It's that simple. Your belief gives your program power, which, in turn, stimulates your body to marshal its own healing resources. There is no better proof of this idea than the abundant scientific evidence proving the power of placebo.

PLACEBO AND THE POWER OF BELIEF

The "placebo effect" refers to a very real and measurable improvement in health that cannot be attributed to any form of medical treatment. It is most often observed when scientists test a particular medication by dividing a cohort of people into two groups: one that gets the active drug and another that gets a pill with no medicinal properties (usually made of sugar or starch), also known as a placebo. The group that gets the real drug is called the experimental group. The group that receives the placebo is referred to as the control group. Neither group knows whether it is receiving the real drug or the sugar pill. Inevitably, many people in the control group report feeling positive effects after taking what they thought was the active drug but, in fact, was the sugar pill. This positive response is known as the placebo effect.

For those taking the placebo, the real source of the health improvement was their belief in the treatment. This belief evokes and strengthens natural forces of healing, which proves sufficient to overcome their illnesses. This same effect turns up in people who undergo what they believe to be an operation. For example, a group of men who suffered from arthritis of the knee reported complete relief of symptoms after being wheeled into an operating room, anesthetized, and having two small incisions made in the backs of their knees to help convince them that they had indeed been operated on. No such operation had occurred, but years later they continued to report complete restoration of their knees and no recurrence of arthritis pain. Similar effects have been shown in both men and women with angina (pain caused by lack of blood flow to the heart) who underwent a sham operation that involved nothing more than a couple of superficial incisions made in the chest.

"The truth is that the placebo effect is huge," wrote Margaret Talbot in the *New York Times Magazine*. "Anywhere between 35 and 75 percent of patients benefit from taking a dummy pill in studies of new drugs—so huge, in fact, that it should probably be put to conscious use in clinical practice, even if we do not entirely understand how it works."

Placebos are constantly disrupting scientific studies because they oftentimes prove just as effective—and sometimes more effective—than the active drugs they are being compared against. In fact, 30 to 40 percent of any test group will respond to placebo, according to Harvard scientist Dr. Henry Beecher. Other studies have shown that, under certain conditions, the numbers are even higher. Of a group of patients treated with placebo for pain, depression, heart disease, gastric ulcers, or asthma, as many as 50 to 60 percent responded positively to placebo. Dr. Irving Kirsch, a psychologist and researcher at the University of Connecticut, believes that up to 75 percent of the effectiveness of Prozac and similar anti-depression drugs may be attributed to placebo. "The critical factor is our belief about what's going to happen to us," Dr. Kirsch told the *New York Times*. "You don't have to rely on drugs to see profound transformation."

Perhaps the placebo effect is nothing more than the use of an external agent to stimulate the body's own healing forces. This certainly is one of the underlying beliefs of alternative medicine—that given the right conditions, the body can heal itself. And, as Norman Cousins and other observers have noted, these healing forces are strengthened when patients believe in their methods of recovery.

When we consider the positive effects of belief on the human body, one cannot help but feel that humans were designed to be optimistic, to believe—and not only to believe in our abilities to recover but also in a higher power that can and will help us in our times of need. This idea leads us to yet another mystery of life that science can observe and document but cannot explain: the healing powers of prayer and meditation.

PRAYER AND MEDITATION

From a purely pragmatic standpoint, prayer and meditation make good sense in recovery because both have been shown to have profoundly positive effects on health. Scientists from UCLA and other university research centers have found that the daily practice of Transcendental Meditation (TM)—in which the person meditating quietly or silently repeats a single word, or mantra, over and over again—reduces blood pressure, atherosclerosis, and incidents of heart attack and stroke.

Daily meditation has been shown to significantly boost the immune system. A study done on men with HIV showed that those who meditated daily experienced an increase in the number and aggressiveness of CD4 cells, the class of immune cells that direct the system's attack against a pathogen. Under normal circumstances, men with HIV experience a steady decline in this essential class of immune cells, but in this study, the men who meditated daily were less likely to see their HIV infection escalate to full-blown AIDS.

Similarly, a study done on medical school students showed that daily meditation or relaxation exercises increased the number and aggressiveness of both natural killer cells and CD4 cells. Other research has shown that daily meditation or relaxation techniques can reduce anxiety and alleviate mild depression.

Harvard Medical School professor Dr. Herbert Benson, famed for his study of the effects of prayer and meditation, has famously suggested that all these effects stem from what he calls the "relaxation response." Dr. Benson's research has shown that ten to twenty minutes of meditation each day can lower blood pressure, slow heart rate, balance hormones, relax muscles, and boost immune function. "Any practice that can evoke the relaxation response is of benefit, be it meditation, yoga, breathing or repetitive prayer," states Dr. Benson. "There is no reason to believe that one [method] is better than the other. The key is the repetition, but the repetition can be a word, sound, mantra, prayer, breathing or movement." According to Dr. Benson, "[j]ust about any condition that is either caused or made worse by stress can be helped with meditation."

Furthermore, prayer has been associated not only with widespread improvements in health but also with miraculous cures that defy scientific explanation. Evidence clearly shows that prayer has the power to heal.

Distant Prayer

"Who has not, during a time of illness or pain, cried out to a higher being for help and healing?" Dr. Randolph Byrd, a professor of medicine at the University of California, San Francisco, asks in the introduction to his study "Positive Therapeutic Effects of Intercessory Prayer in a Coronary Care Unit Population," published in the *Southern Medical Journal*. "Praying for help and healing is a fundamental concept in practically all societies, though the object to which these prayers are directed varies among the religions of the world."

Dr. Byrd was among the first to document scientifically the power of prayer to promote healing. He and his colleagues divided into two groups 393 patients who had recently undergone heart surgery. The first group was composed of 192 patients, each of whom would be prayed for by a member of a local church of Protestant or Roman Catholic denomination. Each person who had agreed to pray was given a patient's first name, diagnosis, and condition, as well as regular updates on that patient's health. At the same time, 201 patients would not be prayed for. These patients would act as the control group. At the outset of the experiment, there were no statistical differences in health between those who would be prayed for and those who would not. The patients did not know that anyone would be prayed for, nor did the scientists know who would be prayed for and who would not.

After nine months, the researchers found that the patients who had been prayed for had also experienced much more rapid healing and far less need for medical intervention than the control group. Those who had been prayed for had seen fewer incidences of congestive heart failure, cardiopulmonary arrest, and pneumonia, and had required less medication and high-tech support than the controls. On the other hand, "[t]he control group had required more ventilatory assistance, antibiotics, and diuretics" than the [prayer] group," according to Dr. Byrd and his colleagues, who concluded, "These data suggest that intercessory prayer to the Judeo-Christian God has a beneficial therapeutic effect in patients admitted to a CCU."

Other studies have found similar effects from distant prayer. Perhaps the most impressive of these was done in 1998 by Duke University scientists. The researchers studied the effects of distant prayer on 150 people who had had invasive cardiac operations. The researchers compared those who were prayed for against a control group composed of people who had undergone the same kinds of procedures but were not the focus of a specific prayer group. The researchers asked seven religious groups to pray for the 150 participants of the experimental group. Those seven religious denominations included Carmelite nuns from Baltimore, a Buddhist group in Nepal, and Virtual Jerusalem, an organization that prays for people upon request and inserts written prayers into the Wailing Wall. As with Dr. Byrd's study, none of the participants knew of the prayers, nor did the scientists themselves know who was being prayed for and who wasn't. The study found that those who had been prayed for had experienced nearly one-third fewer adverse outcomes, such as heart failure, post-procedural ischemia, repeat angioplasty, or heart attack, compared with the control group.

It Just Works

Dr. Harold Koenig, professor of medicine and psychiatry at Duke University, reviewed more than 1,200 scientific studies on prayer and discovered the following:

■ The average hospital stay for hospitalized people who had never attended church was three times longer than those who attended church regularly.

■ Heart patients were fourteen times more likely to die following surgery if they did not participate in a religion.

■ Elderly people who never or rarely attended church had twice the rate of stroke than those who attended church regularly.

■ In Israel, religious people had a 40-percent lower death rate from cardiovascular disease and cancer.

■ People who participated in religion tended to become depressed less often than those who did not, and they also recovered faster from depression when this condition struck.

The crucial factor in these studies may not be a physical appearance at church or synagogue services, per se, but rather the sincere effort to set aside time to pray and connect to whatever you perceive as a Supreme Being. It is this relationship that gives prayer its power. "No problem is too hard for God to solve," writes Marianne Williamson in her book *Everyday Grace*. "This is very important to remember, as it's hard to have deep faith in a kinda-sorta-powerful God."

Mona's Story

When I first met Mona Schwartz she was forty-six years old, the mother of two children, and very much the picture of good health. She had beautiful red hair, large dark blue eyes, and a strong, wide mouth that revealed a radiant, energetic smile. She stood five feet three inches tall and had a slim figure. When the two of us sat down to discuss her own healing journey, Mona produced an array of photographs, most of them of her children, of whom she was obviously very proud. She then showed me a photograph of herself, or, I should say, her former self, which at first I had difficulty believing could be her.

The picture was of Mona standing on the deck of a boat, wearing a raincoat that was bursting from her girth. She weighed more than 170 pounds. Her stomach was so distended that it looked like she was carrying a beach ball under her raincoat. At the time, Mona also suffered from a litany of severe illnesses, including acute thyroid, kidney, gall bladder, and liver disorders; toxemia; idiopathic edema; severe back and neck pain; and chronic diarrhea. She had already undergone numerous surgeries and was taking a plethora of medications. Recent blood tests had revealed the possibility of cancer of the liver, but her doctors needed to do a biopsy to know for sure.

Mona was from Philadelphia and her biopsy was to be done at Graduate Hospital. On the night before the surgery, Mona walked the halls of the hospital, despondent. She decided that she didn't care if she lived or died—life had become too much for her to bear. Soon, Mona found herself in a poorly lit, silent, empty corridor. Tall windows were on both sides of the hall, but outside, the world was dark. Suddenly, a strange light appeared directly in front of her. The apparition asked Mona if she wanted to live. Deeply stirred, Mona fell to her knees and said, "I want to live, God. I want to live." Her words were met with silence.

The following morning Mona underwent biopsy surgery, which revealed that there was no cancer in her liver. After the operation, she was returned to her room. As she gradually regained consciousness, Mona heard the words come from deep within: "Then you shall live." A week later, she adopted a diet and lifestyle that would help her regain her health.

Mona's story exemplifies the experience of being led by spiritual forces to a practical, down-to-earth solution for which prayers were uttered. Even before she was led to a solution, something within Mona had already been transformed. She had surrendered in faith, and thus could be led to her answer. And when it was presented, she could accept and follow the guidance offered.

When it comes to faith, we must walk along its path believing that we are being led to our solutions, and at the same time we must constantly assess if our programs are working and yielding practical results. Such faith is an essential part of the healing process. If you develop and sustain your faith, there will be tangible—even undeniable—signs along the way to show you that you are either on the right track or the wrong one. You must keep your eyes, ears, and heart open. On the practical side, your program should positively affect your medical tests, including your blood values. Other signs of progress may include improvements in your energy levels, weight, sleep, mood, and many important physical functions, such as digestion and elimination.

As you pray, meditate, or engage in other spiritual pursuits, events will likely occur that open your heart and mind to the possibility that something larger than yourself is guiding you. You may experience mysterious coincidences that turn out to be life-changing. You may meet people who seem destined to play a part in your life. A new world will start to open up to you, one that can only be described as spiritual in nature.

What Lies Beneath

We don't typically turn to science for a better understanding of such phenomena, but our understanding of the relationship between certain sciences and spirituality is changing. Increasingly, physicists are finding that the material universe, based on the old Newtonian physics, is but a shell of a much larger set of mysteries that lie below. The fact is that all physical matter is composed of energy. Sub atomic particles, the very building blocks of matter, when looked at more closely, are nothing more than pure energy with no solidity at all. Quantum physicist Dr. Fred Alan Wolf explains it this way: We are taught to believe that matter is composed of atoms, which are like "itsy-bitsy baseballs." Yet, when you look closer at these tiny particles, "the little baseballs do not behave like little baseballs—they refract or bend and spread out like waves, producing wave patterns."

We are so familiar with the material world and its obvious rules—one should not walk into the path of large, moving objects, for example—that we forget there is another side of life, a world of energy beneath the surface of material existence. When science looks below the surface of ordinary reality, another universe reveals itself, one that offers miraculous potential.

"At the quantum level, nothing of the material world is left intact," writes Deepak Chopra in his book *How to Know God*. "It is strange enough to hold up your hand and realize that it is actually, at a deeper level, invisible vibrations taking place in a void. . . . At the quantum level the whole cosmos is like a blinking light. There are no stars or galaxies, only vibrating energy fields that our senses are too dull and slow to pick up given the incredible speed at which light and electricity move." This is the paradoxical world in which we live—at the surface, solid to the touch, but below, nothing but moving waves. Each of these conditions offers us a very different set of possibilities. In material reality, we need tangible food, live in houses that protect us against the elements, and drive cars to traverse long distances. At the material level, prayer makes no sense at all because everything is separate and there is nothing visible that might unify anything, much less each of us. But at the quantum level, prayer makes complete sense because all material reality originates from energy; everything is made of energy; and everything is influenced by it. Since prayer is essentially directed thought and emotion—which are waves of energy—it can reach anything and anyone in the quantum field, where all things are unified.

Do you acknowledge both sides of reality, or do you focus on one side over the other? According to Dr. Wolf, "[t]he universe can appear to be fundamentally paradoxical. . . . The more we determine one side of reality, the less the other side is shown to us."

Chopra offers a simple metaphor to show how these apparent opposites may be reconciled so that we may better understand our relationship with God. He states that reality is like a three-layer sandwich. The first layer is the material world, bound by all the laws of Newtonian physics. At this level, there appear to be no phenomena that cannot be explained through rational science. Indeed, all rational arguments against the existence of God seem entirely persuasive.

The top layer of the sandwich is what we refer to as God. And in between, there is a transitional zone where "God and humans meet on common ground." According to Chopra, this is where "miracles take place, along with holy visions, angels, enlightenment, and hearing the voice of God. All of this extraordinary phenomena bridge two worlds: They are real and yet they are not part of a predictable cause-and-effect."

The quantum dimension is the transitional zone where energy becomes matter. To put it another way, quantum reality is the dimension where thoughts, emotions, behavior, and prayers (all in the form of energy) change the quality of our health (matter)—and even the health of people at great distances. As inhabitants of quantum reality, we can call upon this power to turn energy into matter, or to make our hopes and prayers reality. This is where belief and faith come into the picture. People may insist that reality is based on rational, material laws, and they have good reasons to think they're right. But as quantum physicists point out, if you insist on seeing only one side of reality, that is the reality you will get, and the one you will be forced to live.

The Strongest Belief Wins

Physicists point out that the quantum realm is made up of infinite energy, and as such, it is the dimension of pure potential. The waves in the quantum field are waiting to be organized and bundled into specific forms of matter and new experiences in everyday life. The mechanism by which potential energy in the quantum field becomes matter or events is through the power of our daily thoughts, emotions, and behaviors. You create your own reality through the kinds of thoughts, emotions, expectations, and behaviors you engage in every day. In the world of pure potential, positive thoughts, prayers, chants, and meditations—when focused on specific goals, images, or conditions—have the power to organize infinite energy and create new realities. "This means that the quantum field contains a reality in which you are healthy, wealthy, and happy, and possess all the qualities and capabilities of the idealized self that you hold in your thoughts," writes Dr. Joe Dispenza in his book *Breaking the Habit of Being Yourself*. "Like clay, the energy of infinite possibilities is shaped by consciousness: your mind," writes Dr. Dispenza.

But there's the rub. The quantum field responds to your strongest beliefs, which possess the most powerful thought waves. So, if you're trying to manifest one belief but, in fact, actually believe more strongly in another, the stronger belief will win. This is why so many spiritual traditions and teachers recommend consistency in daily prayer and meditation practice. Positive beliefs become stronger with practice. Your confidence, perhaps once small and overwhelmed by doubt, may grow. Little by little, your faith can tip the balance in favor of the miraculous.

But there is more going on than simply the power of our own thoughts to shape reality. To go back to Chopra's metaphor—the reality sandwich— our rational intellect cannot perceive anything beyond the material world, which thus undermines both our faith and the power of prayer. But with regular prayer and meditation, we start to connect to larger spiritual larger forces in the universe, which respond by offering us clues to their presence. Among the most common of such clues is the experience of unexplainable coincidences and tangible improvements in health. These subtle—and sometimes not-so-subtle—forms of correspondence awaken in us the feeling of being helped by powers greater than our own.

"Each of us can live in the victory of spirit, claiming for ourselves the miraculous power that has been given to us as children of God," writes Marianne Williamson in *Everyday Grace*. "It is in our *faith* that miracles are possible—that the very fabric of the universe is miraculous—which opens the mind, and thus the future, to unimaginable possibilities. 'Dear God, please send a miracle' is a powerful prayer for cosmic support. To pray is to take spiritual action."

Often, when we look back on the healing journey we have traveled, it is with awe, for events occur that baffle the mind and leave us speechless with wonder. This was certainly the case for Dr. Anthony Sattilaro, who was dying from prostate cancer and desperate for a miracle.

Where Medicine and Spirituality Become One

On June 1, 1978, doctors at Methodist Hospital in Philadelphia, Pennsylvania, informed Dr. Anthony Sattilaro that he had prostate cancer that had spread throughout his body. In addition to the cancer in his prostate, x-rays and bone scans had revealed tumors in his skull, spine, sternum, left sixth rib, and right shoulder. Dr. Sattilaro, who was then president of Methodist Hospital, was told that he had approximately one year to eighteen months left to live. He was forty-eight years old. Prostate cancer in men younger than fifty is a highly virulent and lethal disease. He did an exhaustive investigation of his illness and sought counsel from medical experts across the country, all of whom agreed that he had little chance of recovery.

In order to give him as much time as possible, doctors surgically removed Dr. Sattilaro's left sixth rib, which was full of cancer, and both of his testicles. The latter procedure was done to reduce his testosterone levels, which can fuel prostate cancer and make it spread more rapidly. Dr. Sattilaro was also given therapeutic estrogens in the hope that the drugs would also slow the cancer. These approaches did not have any real impact on his disease, but they did cause significant side effects, including profuse itching, intense nausea, and vomiting. Dr. Sattilaro's body became bloated and overweight. The five-foot-six-inch man soon weighed 170 pounds—25 pounds above his normal, healthy weight.

The tumors in his spine caused him tremendous pain for which he was taking an array of powerful analgesics, including Percodan. Unfortunately, the drugs tended to wear off long before he could safely take another dosage, which meant that each day he was forced to endure many hours of agonizing pain. While this was going on, Dr. Sattilaro's father was dying of lung cancer. As he watched his father wither away, he realized that he himself would soon follow in his father's footsteps. On August 7, 1978, Dr. Sattilaro's father died.

After the funeral, which was held in New Jersey, Dr. Sattilaro drove back to Philadelphia. On the highway going home, he spotted two hitchhikers by the side of the road and decided to pick them up. It was uncharacteristic of him to do such a thing. What made him do it is anyone's guess. He stopped and let Sean McLean and Bill Bochbracher enter his car—McLean in front, Bochbracher in back. The two travelers were on their way to North Carolina to study cooking. They were affable young men, both in their mid-twenties. Soon Bachbracher went to sleep and eventually Dr. Sattilaro told McLean that he had just buried his father, who had died of cancer, and that he himself was dying of cancer. The next words that came from McLean's mouth have come to be famous in certain circles of natural healing. To be sure, they would change Dr. Sattilaro's life, as well as tens of thousands of other lives, thanks to a bestselling book entitled *Recalled By Life*, which Dr. Sattilaro would go on to write.

"You don't have to die, doc. Cancer isn't all that hard to cure," the young cook said. Dr. Sattilaro was utterly offended. Years later, he reflected on McLean's comment. "I looked at him and thought, 'this is just a silly kid.' Here I was a doctor for 20 years. I knew that cancer was very difficult to cure, and we didn't have the answers." McLean, a student of macrobiotics, insisted that a macrobiotic diet and way of life could restore Dr. Sattilaro's health. He pressed him to drive to Essene Natural Foods Store in Philadelphia, where he might meet the local macrobiotic teacher, a man named Denny Waxman. Dr. Sattilaro took McLean and Bochbracher to Essene, but Waxman was out. Reluctantly, Mclean and Bochbracher left the doctor and resumed their travels, but not before they got his address. Two weeks later, a large manila envelope arrived at Dr. Sattilaro's door. The envelope, sent from McLean, contained a booklet entitled *A Macrobiotic Approach to Cancer*. Dr. Sattilaro gave the thing a perfunctory perusal and was about to toss it in the wastebasket when his eye caught the name of a Philadelphia physician whose written testimonial described the use of a macrobiotic diet in her treatment of cancer. He looked up the physician's name in a medical directory and telephoned her at home. A man answered. Dr. Sattilaro explained the reason he was calling and asked for the woman.

"I'm sorry," the man said. "My wife isn't here. She's in the hospital dying of cancer."

"Oh, I see," Dr. Sattilaro replied. "Well, you've answered my question. Macrobiotics doesn't cure cancer." With that, he was about to hang up when the man answered with enthusiasm. "Listen, it really works," he said. "While she was sticking to the diet, it really did help her. She showed real signs of getting well. But she couldn't stick to it. She hated the food."

"Do you think it's worth looking into?" Dr. Sattilaro asked. "I'm dying of cancer."

"Yes, definitely," the man replied.

The next call Dr. Sattilaro made was to Denny Waxman. The two met soon thereafter at Denny's home in a suburb of Philadelphia. Denny Waxman, then thirty years of age, was lean, healthy-looking, and serious. Waxman gave Dr. Sattilaro a very strange examination in which he looked carefully at Satillaro's face, arms, feet, and the sclera (white part) of each of his eyes. Once he completed his examination, Waxman outlined the diet he wanted Dr. Sattilaro to eat. It was composed of cooked whole grains, fresh vegetables, beans, sea vegetables, and soup that contained miso, a base made from fermented soybeans. The diet also included a variety of condiments and some seeds and nuts. Waxman said that when Dr. Sattilaro became stronger, he could include fish and some fruit, but until he showed real signs of improvement, he should abstain from these foods. After he finished describing the diet, Waxman encouraged Dr. Sattilaro, saying that he had a strong constitution and a good chance of recovery. "What the hell," Dr. Sattilaro told himself as he left Denny Waxman's house that day. "I'm going to die anyway, so I might as well give this diet a try."

Dr. Sattilaro did not cook—he ate all his meals in restaurants—and after a few valiant but failed attempts at cooking in the kitchen, he accepted Denny's invitation to eat his meals at the Waxman table. There he learned about macrobiotics. It was not a subject that gave him all that much peace. He soon found that the world of macrobiotics was more than simply a diet or nutritional approach to illness and health. Rather, it was a philosophical approach to living.

Unlike modern science, ancient, traditional medical systems such as macrobiotics combine practical healing arts with a philosophy about the underlying life force that animates the body and is the basis for health. Virtually all traditional healing systems were founded on such a philosophy, including the Greek (in which life force is called "pneuma," or breath), Hindu (in which life force is called "prana"), and Chinese (in which the life force is called "qi"). Belief in a life force is also present in Judaism and early Christianity. In these traditions, life force is linked to spirit, which refers to one's own individual spirit and the larger life force that permeates the universe.

This animating life force is strengthened, according to macrobiotic philosophy, when two opposing forces—one contracting, the other expanding—are brought into balance. These forces are known as yin and yang. A plant-based diet, free of refined foods, artificial ingredients, and sugar, is one of the primary tools for bringing these forces into harmony, and thus the foundation for restoring and maintaining health.

Dr. Sattilaro's medical training had given him a scientific, materialistic outlook on life. He had come to believe that if you couldn't see the object in question, or measure it with a machine, it didn't exist. Hence, he thought macrobiotic ideas were ludicrous. "When I came to Denny's house," he recalled years later, "I thought that this was the biggest bunch of weirdoes I'd ever seen. They were all sitting [Japanese-style] on the floor, ready to eat with chopsticks. Then they started to pray and I just thought that this was a bunch of crap."

The only potentially valuable idea in macrobiotics that he could discern was the relationship between food and health. The belief that excessive consumption of meat, eggs, chicken, dairy products, sugar, and processed foods caused disease made sense to him. At least that was something he could rationalize. He strongly doubted that a macrobiotic diet could reverse his illness, but he had to eat, and plant foods were clearly nutritious. It would be a far healthier diet than the one he had been following.

There was, however, something that kept him coming back to macrobiotics. On an intuitive level, he felt what he was doing was right. He couldn't articulate the source of his feeling. Yet, his gut urged him on. So, every evening he returned to the Waxman table and ate this very strange food with his chopsticks. After dinner, Denny's wife, Judy, sent Dr. Sattilaro off with additional food for breakfast and lunch the following day. Despite his skepticism, he made a complete commitment and followed the diet with absolute strictness. Anything Denny recommended, he did. The diet was the only thing that gave him hope, and he would not weaken his chances of recovery by being self-indulgent. It wasn't long before his diligence was rewarded.

On the morning of September 26, just one month after he had met Denny Waxman, Dr. Sattilaro got out of bed, reached for his pain killer (in this case Percodan), and, still half asleep, suddenly realized the pain in his back was gone. He jumped out of bed and searched his back with his mind. Still nothing. He walked around his bedroom and did some gentle stretching. Gone. Not a trace of pain could be found in his back or anywhere else in his body. He had been suffering with this agonizing pain for two years. Only the most powerful narcotics could ease it. And now, for reasons he could not understand, the pain had disappeared.

This milestone convinced Dr. Sattilaro that the diet was deeply affecting his health and perhaps his cancer. From there, he began to make steady and, at times, seemingly miraculous progress. His energy levels dramatically improved. His appearance changed. He lost the excess weight, regained a youthful glow in his features, and looked years younger. Soon it became clear to those around him that he was not following the standard path of a man dying of cancer. One of his friends and colleagues, Dr. John Giacobbo, vice president of Methodist Hospital, recalled his progress. "When Tony first started the macrobiotic diet, people thought it was some kind of far-out idea," he said. "Some people at the hospital thought he was a kook. I told him he was crazy. Pretty soon, though, you could see he was improving mentally and physically."

Throughout the fall and winter, Dr. Sattilaro's health continued to improve, and in the spring of 1979, he decided that the therapeutic estrogens he was taking were actually an impediment to his health and recovery. Despite his doctor's strong opposition, Dr. Sattilaro stopped the drugs, and in the weeks and months that followed, his health only got stronger.

Meanwhile, his healing journey led to a spiritual transformation. He went back to his Roman Catholic roots and became deeply involved in the Church. He regularly traveled to monasteries and took part in meditative retreats. He prayed throughout the day—more formally each morning and evening, and in small ways throughout the course of his day. He read spiritual literature voraciously and sought the guidance of clergy. In fact, the macrobiotic experience reinforced many of his fundamental spiritual beliefs. In the process of taking this new approach to healing, he came to see his life's most profound spiritual imbalances.

Dr. Sattilaro realized he had been dominated by the intellectual center of his being and its tendencies to see people and events as separate and distinct from each other and from himself. He now knew that such a point of view, though important in certain contexts, was only a partial understanding of reality. There was another way of seeing things—a more unified approach to life in which all events, all people, all phenomena are united by the web of life, a web that itself might be understood as a living, spiritual entity.

These two points of view give rise to very distinct ways of thinking and behaving, and indeed very different qualities of life. The intellectual view sees people as striving after limited resources, and therefore promotes fear and selfishness. It's a dog-eat-dog world, says the intellectual center. Get what you can and survive. In fact, this was Dr. Sattilaro's way of life prior to getting cancer. He was profoundly ambitious and determined to get all he could for himself. Now he saw clearly that he had to change. As it happened, this change was staring him in the face. It was there in his healing path.

The belief in a universe infused with a life energy that is constantly seeking harmony suggests that life itself is a perfectly coordinated entity in which all people and events are connected. This unified worldview recognizes our commonality, our inherent oneness with the universe and each other. Such a view rejects separation and fear, and embraces unity, compassion, love, and healing. In order to heal himself, Dr. Sattilaro knew he had to change his thinking and his way living to conform to this unified perspective on being, which was essentially positive and optimistic. He had to start believing in the possibility of a miracle.

On September 25, 1979, just sixteen months after his diagnosis, Dr. Sattilaro underwent a bone scan and x-rays, all of which showed no sign of cancer in his body. Those who had watched him go through his healing odyssey were convinced that his macrobiotic approach had restored his health. "Most people at Methodist were convinced that Dr. Sattilaro was going to die. The five-year survival rate for this type of illness is zero. Now, he is completely cured and I'm amazed. I think the diet did it," said Dr. Giacobbo.

Many people argued that Dr. Sattilaro's recovery was some kind of miracle. "Of course it was a miracle," he would reply. "God directed me to pick up Sean McLean and Bill Bochbracher. There's no doubt in my mind that God has been with me every step of the way."

The rest of Dr. Sattilaro's story is meaningful and instructive on many levels. His healing experience became a well-known recovery story, and he received a significant level of attention in the press and on television and radio. As he gained notoriety for his cancer recovery story, his position at Methodist Hospital became increasingly untenable. As he told me after his recovery, "I became a walking reminder of a healing approach that medicine didn't want any part of. People didn't want me around." He was considered an embarrassment to those who insisted that diet had no place in the treatment of cancer. Highly placed physicians predicted he would be dead within two years.

Eventually, Dr. Sattilaro was forced to leave his job and the profession he loved. When he lost his job, he essentially lost his purpose for living. He could not help but draw a parallel to another famous figure that had been raised from the dead. "I was just like Lazarus," he said. "After Lazarus was restored to life, people wanted him dead again, because he was a reminder of Jesus. Many people in my profession wanted me dead, too, because I was a reminder of the role diet could play in healing."

He moved to Florida, fell into depression, and soon gave up his macrobiotic diet. "It took two years of eating fatty foods and sugar for my cancer to return," he said. When it was clear that his cancer was back, he telephoned Michio Kushi, who began counseling him again. In the summer of 1990, Dr. Sattilaro attended the Kushi Institute summer conference at Simon's Rock in Great Barrington, Massachusetts. Before the few hundred people gathered at the conference, he announced that he had twice proved that macrobiotics cured his cancer.

"The first time was when I got cancer and adopted macrobiotics and cured myself," he said. "The second time was when I went off the diet and got the disease back." Later that summer, he died of cancer.

Just as there were numerous factors that led to his recovery, so, too, were there many different components that led to the recurrence of his disease and death. In fact, Dr. Sattilaro proved the seven steps in reverse. As he was pushed out of his job, he became angry, afraid, and depressed. He gave up the diet that had helped him recover. He lost his focus and commitment to the many healing practices he had adopted. He also broke off all contact with the healers and the community that supported his healing. He surrendered his faith and, with the loss of his job, lost his sense of purpose. Once his cancer returned, there was no controlling it, even with all available medical treatment and the resumption of his healing diet.

As we may infer from Dr. Sattilaro's experience, a cascade of destructive events can occur when we lose faith—or, to put it in another way, when we remain under the influence of negative beliefs and emotional states for an extended period of time. Without faith, there is little hope, and without hope, positive action seems pointless. Faith is more than a catalyst for positive action, though; it is also a force—indeed, life energy—that infuses each action with healing power.

Let us consider the possibility that faith is an evolutionary leap beyond mere belief. In belief, there is an intellectual insistence, in large part because belief is always tied to doubt. With belief comes hope, but in hope lies the shadow of uncertainty. As we have seen, belief is essential to the healing process, but it does not have the power of faith. Faith is beyond the dualities that are still present in belief. There is in faith a deep knowing that is not of the mind but of the heart. In the beginning of our healing process, we maintain, as best we can, a belief in recovery. But as we proceed along this path, events occur that awaken us to the subtle clues that we are being loved and led. We follow the path with a heart that is more open. We develop faith.

WHAT TO DO NOW

Prayers can be as simple as clearly stating your request, or as elaborate as reciting favorite passages from sacred literature or the prayers you were taught as a child. Two ideas, however, are of paramount importance regarding prayer. First, we are instructed by many religious traditions to pray continuously throughout the day. A wonderful short volume entitled *The Practice of the Presence of God*, written by Brother Lawrence, a French monk who lived in the seventeenth century, instructs us merely to talk to God on an ongoing basis throughout the day. Brother Lawrence says that you should treat God as if God were at your side as you walk through life. As you walk with God, share all your thoughts, emotions, fears, and desires.

Turn all that you are burdened by over to Him. This, says Brother Lawrence, is the practice of the presence of God. As he wrote to a fellow member of the clergy in 1682, "There is no manner of life in the world more sweet or more delicious than continual conversation with God. They alone can understand it who practice it and savor it. . . . Believe me; make a holy and firm resolve never voluntarily to withdraw yourself from God's grace from this time on. Live the rest of your days in God's holy presence. . . . "

The second important step, especially as it relates to health, is to pray until you feel relief from your fears and anxiety. As you begin, you may feel overwhelmed by both these feelings. Keep praying until they pass and you experience a degree of serenity and protection.

As you pray, concentrate on your image of the Divine, a holy figure, a patron saint, or an ancestor who loved you and watched over you while he or she was alive. You may instead want to concentrate on the image of a sacred light, which many believe is the closest image we have of God. Whatever the symbol, try to communicate all that you feel. Relax into its embrace and feel your communion with it. As you pray, your emotions will begin to change. You may simply experience relief from your fear. You may experience anger or even sadness. Keep praying. As mentioned, anger can eventually lead to sadness, which can release so much emotion. Let it come out. Sadness is a gateway to compassion for yourself and others. Once you feel compassion for yourself, you may want to stop praying now and simply feel the emotions rise through your body and heart. Feel the love you have for yourself and others. Sit with those feelings and allow them to comfort you.

As Dr. Benson says, it doesn't matter whether you pray or meditate; what matters is that you say the words over and over again until you achieve what he calls the "relaxation response." Here are some suggestions for prayers, meditations, and chants that can inspire strength and hope.

Praying

In addition to the following prayer suggestions, I have also provided a list of organizations that, upon request, will pray for you. The addresses and other contact information of these organizations can be found in the Resources section (see page 217) of this book.

■ Engage in repetitive prayer, such as chanting, saying the Rosary, or davening (performing the Jewish recitation prayers). These practices evoke the relaxation response and have the power to take us beyond our anxieties and fears into a state of calm and peace.

■ Pray directly to God, or to a holy figure, such as Jesus, Moses, Buddha, or the Divine Mother, however you conceive of any of these beings. Pray in the morning, during the day, and at night. Prayer can be especially powerful whenever we feel anxious or afraid.

■ A very simple, yet powerful spiritual practice is to read a chapter a day from either the Jewish or Christian Bible. If you do this practice consistently, you very likely will experience a profound transformation in your feelings about yourself, your life, and your relationship with God. Consistent reading of the Bible promotes strong belief and deep faith in the God's love.

■ Read passages or chapters from other sacred literature, such as the Bhagavad Gita, the Sutras of Shakyamuni Buddha, the Vedas and the Uphanisads, or the Koran.

■ Read inspirational books that touch your heart and soul and make you feel closer to the Divine.

In *The Power of Positive Thinking,* Norman Vincent Peale tells the story of a former major league baseball pitcher, Frank Hiller, who pitched a complete nine-inning game in temperatures that were well in excess of 100°F. In the process, he lost several pounds and at one point his energy began to flag badly. In a very short period, however, his strength returned and he appeared to grow stronger as the game progressed. Asked after the game how he had pulled off such a feat, he told a reporter that he had repeated a phrase from the Old Testament over and over again: "But they that wait upon the Lord shall renew their strength; they shall mount up with wings as eagles, they shall run, and not be weary; and they shall walk and not faint." (Isaiah 40:31). Every time he had said these words, he had felt himself getting stronger. "I passed a powerful energy-producing thought through my mind," he said.

As Peale says, "Contact with God establishes within us a flow of the same type of energy that re-creates the world and that renews springtime every year. When in spiritual contact with God through our thought processes, the Divine energy flows through the personality, automatically renewing the original creative act. When contact with the Divine energy is broken, the personality gradually becomes depleted in body, mind, and spirit. An electric clock connected with an outlet does not run down and will continue indefinitely to keep accurate time. Unplug it, and the clock stops. It has lost contact with the power flowing through the universe."

Many people feel more comfort during prayer when they create an altar in their homes. An altar can be a low table upon which you can place spiritual articles that inspire your reverence for the sacred. Of course, the altar should be set up in a very private place in your home—a quiet corner of your bedroom, for example, or a room that does not get much traffic. This altar will become the outward symbol and a reminder of the sacred in your life. Whether you create an altar or not, it's important to pray in a quiet setting that will allow you to go deeply inside yourself and encourage your feelings to emerge.

Pray for Others and Ask Others to Pray for You

Every church, synagogue, and temple offers community prayers to those who are suffering from illness or some other difficult circumstance. Ask your local religious community to include you in their prayers. If you do not have a local religious community, there are many religious-based groups that will pray for you. Among them are the Carmelite nuns, which have monasteries throughout the world. The Carmelite nuns, an order of cloistered Catholic nuns, will pray for anyone in need of help. Virtual Jerusalem, an Internet organization of Jewish people, also accepts prayer requests from anyone. In addition, there are many Protestant sects that accept requests for prayers on an ongoing basis. Addresses for these and other organizations can be found in the Resources section (see page 217) of this book.

If you have a close-knit group of friends who are spiritually oriented, ask your friends to form a prayer support group. Moreover, pray for others who need help. Your prayers for others who are suffering can strengthen you and awaken you to your power to help others in their healing. All spiritual practices, no matter what their religious source, should bring you back into an intimate and loving relationship with yourself and with your perception of God. Spiritual practice is the act of attuning your awareness to your heart and soul—the most essential aspects of self. So many people who became ill have told me that somewhere along the way they lost track of themselves. The demands of their lives overtook them. Life sped up and got out of control. In the course of things, they found themselves relating more to the demands of the world than to the subtle urges of their inner lives. This, they say, is how they lost connection with themselves. Prayer can bring you back into connection with yourself and all that is important in your life.

Chanting

Science tells us that energy proceeds matter and thus gives birth to matter, which means that thoughts and words—as forms of energy—can have great power that can shape the reality of your inner world and dramatically affect your outer life. Each thought and word is imbued with a frequency that affects your individual cells and overall physical body. As everyone knows, words of love can open your heart and transform how you feel, not just because of their associations but also because of the immensely powerful frequencies that are implicit within words of love. These frequencies uplift, energize, and inspire. They breathe life into cells.

Listen or recite poetry. Read a great speech. Listen to great music. These expressions of love can, in a matter of seconds, transform your respiration, making it deeper and more rhythmic; change your hormonal balance and diminish the level of stress hormones coursing through your bloodstream; and alter your brain chemistry, and thus release layers of physical tension.

Throughout human history, people have chanted powerful prayers to uplift their minds and hearts and to elevate the frequencies of their bodies in order to transcend the intellectual realm. Chanting, or the singing of prayers, can be a powerful and transformative practice that can have a soothing, relaxing, and healing effect on your body, mind, emotional life, and spirit. There are many powerful chants you can use. You can purchase CDs or digital recordings for all types of chanting, including Christian, Gregorian, Sufi, Hindu, Buddhist, and Jewish prayers and songs. Among the words most commonly chanted is "Om," which, in the Hindu tradition, is the sacred sound of the universe. It is widely believed that when you chant this sound again and again, you align yourself with the rhythm and the energy of the core of the universe, or God. Chanting Om creates for many a deep state of reverence, relaxation, and meditation. For those who have trouble emptying their minds during meditation, chanting Om can free you of much distress, anxiety, and excessive thinking.

"Nam Myoho Renge Kyo" is a Buddhist chant that means devotion to the mystic law of cause and effect through sound. It is believed by some Buddhist sects to be the most powerful and transformative sound one can make. Many Buddhists believe that Nam Myoho Renge Kyo causes the Buddha nature—the most advanced form of consciousness implicit in all people—to come into being and take hold of our ordinary, everyday judgment. The chant opens the spiritual channel that runs down the center of the body, boosting the life force to every cell and fiber of the body and spirit.

Nam Myoho Renge Kyo is one of the most physically and spiritually empowering chants ever created. Try chanting it slowly or rapidly and rhythmically and see what effects it has on your physical and emotional states of being.

An ancient Japanese chant is "Su," a sound that is designed to open the heart. Another ancient chant is a derivation of Om, "A-U-M," which is designed to send loving, healing energies to three energy centers of your body—the pelvis, the region of your heart and upper chest, and finally your neck and head. The sound "A" is pronounced "ahh" and is intended to direct energy to deep into your bladder, reproductive organs, and pelvic region. As you say the "ahh" sound, see if you can't direct the vibration down into your lower belly and pelvis. The "U" is pronounced as a soft "ooohhh." The vibration is meant to be concentrated in your chest and heart. The "M" sound vibrates most acutely in your head and throat. Chant all three sounds—"A-U-M"—and feel the vibration shift from lower, to middle, to higher as you chant each of the three syllables. This chant grounds you deeply in your body and autonomic nervous system, the branch of the nervous system that runs to your heart, abdomen, lower belly, and pelvis. It will reduce excessive thinking and allow you to feel centered and balanced in your body.

Chanting is incredibly energizing and strengthening. Choose any sound to which you have a heartfelt connection and chant it throughout the day. You can chant a sacred sound quietly to yourself, or out loud in the privacy of your home or a peaceful natural environment, such as a forest or seashore.

Meditation

Meditation is literally the training of your mind. Just as you would train your body to better perform a particular task, such a sport or a musical instrument, meditation trains the mind to become more stable and experience greater clarity, insight, and happiness. Consciousness is layered. Love, wisdom, beauty, and happiness exist deep within us all. Unfortunately, at the more superficial layers of awareness, more negative states prevail, including fear, anger, anxiety, jealousy, greed, hatred, and violence. Meditation silences and stabilizes the mind so that negative emotions dissipate and clear, allowing the deeper layers of love, wisdom, and clarity to emerge. This is one of the reasons why meditation is associated with improvements in health. A meditation practice frees the mind from the very causes of illness—various forms of stress, fear, anger, hatred, and greed, all of which destroy both the mind and the body. Conversely, states of beauty, love, and wisdom are inherently healing. As these occupy the mind, they change the way the body functions, promoting health and well-being.

There are many forms of meditation. Among the oldest, simplest, and most powerful meditation techniques is the act of sitting peacefully and concentrating on your breath. This meditative tool can be used in a quiet setting, such as your home, but also at any time of day, even in the most crowded of rooms or stressful of situations. It will immediately bring about feelings of greater calm and self-control. This meditation itself is utterly simple yet so engaging and demanding that you could spend a lifetime developing your ability to practice it.

Begin the meditation by placing both feet on the floor. Place your hands comfortably in your lap and drop your shoulders. Focus all your attention on your breathing—concentrate on your breath as you inhale. Concentrate on the small pause at the end of your inhalation. As you exhale, keep your focus on your breath and the long pause at the end of your exhalation. Continue breathing, and as you do, continue concentrating on this simple, rhythmic action that sustains your life. Every time your mind wanders, bring your attention back to your breath. Relax. Breathe. As you focus on your breath, allow the tension to drain from your body. Envision the muscles in your lower back and pelvis relaxing. Feel yourself sinking ever more deeply into your body. Each inhalation becomes a tool for receiving life energy; each exhalation becomes a way to release layers of tension from your body.

As you do this meditation, your mind will quickly quiet. When thoughts arise, observe them without engaging them. You are an objective witness, an observer, to whatever your mind may conjure up or present to you. As much as possible, do not engage your thoughts, anxiety, or fears. They are merely clouds passing gently before you. Let the wind take them where it will.

Memories and emotions may rise as you do this exercise. Observe them with the same dispassion. Your body is an enormous vase that contains many thoughts, emotions, and memories. As you relax and watch your breath, your body will try to release these mental images. They create tension and fear in your body and contribute to your illness. Let them go. Let your body cleanse itself. When your mind wanders, bring your concentration back to your breath. When a thought or memory or emotion rises, it will try to pull you into its drama. Observe it as it rises and fades away. Do not judge anything that comes up. Don't get hooked by it. Don't fight it.

Don't repress it. Allow it to rise, appear before your mind's eye, and then fade away. Come back to your breath. If you find yourself engaging in any thought, memory, or emotion, come back to your breath. Don't engage in any recrimination of yourself. Exhale. Watch your breath. You will get better at this practice over time. Eventually, you will come to a state of deep relaxation and calm. With time, you will get so good at this that you will want to stay here for as long as possible.

Guided Imagery

Watch your breath until you are relaxed and centered. When you feel sufficiently relaxed, imagine a small diamond of light suddenly appearing in the area of your heart. Observe this light and notice that it is extremely powerful and determined. Realize that this is a living entity that is connected to an infinite source of energy. It has the purest, most loving of intentions. It has come to help you. As you observe this light, see it slowly growing larger. See the center of this light and its radiant beams expanding. Feel this light filling your heart with a warm sensation of love, joy, and peace. Allow it to grow and fill your entire chest with these same healing sensations.

Picture a powerful beam of light growing from the bottom of this living energy in your heart and moving into your stomach, intestinal area, and pelvis. Feel it permeating every cell in your digestive tract, abdomen, reproductive organs, and pelvis. Feel its healing energy reaching every inch of your lower body. Recognize that no cell is left in the dark. All are alive and strengthened with this healing energy of light. All the tension in your lower body is giving way to this light. Any obstruction must break up and dissolve before its overwhelming power. See the darkness and blockages break up and fade into the atmosphere outside your body. See every diseased cell either being restored to the light or dying instantly.

From the center of your chest, picture another beam of light growing upward and spreading healing energy to your shoulders, armpits, neck, and head. Feel it infusing your entire upper body with light that overcomes all darkness, all tension, and all resistance. Feel it permeating your entire nervous system, every cell and fiber of your upper body. See the light filling your head with love and compassion. Picture the light moving from your armpits into your arms and hands, again filling every cell with healing energy. See it bursting forth from your fingertips. See it moving from your pelvis and reproductive organs to your thighs, knees, calves, ankles, and feet, filling every cell and then bursting forth from your toes.

Picture your entire body infused with light, love, and healing energy. See the light growing beyond the boundaries of your body so that you find yourself sitting in a ball of light and love. Notice that the light that engulfs your body is now radiating outward and joining an enormous source of energy just above your head. Know that the energy that imbues your body is joined to an infinite source of unconditional love and healing energy that is being channeled into you. See your heart welcoming this abundant energy and distributing it throughout your body, especially to those places that need it most. Bathe in this energy and the love, warmth, and compassion with which it is holding you. Use your breath to direct the energy to any place that it is needed. Relax and sit in this energy until you are ready to emerge from the meditation.

Meditation does not have to be long or drawn out. Give whatever time you can to it—five or ten minutes may be all that is needed, especially in the beginning of your practice, to give you a sense of peace, comfort, and connection to the larger life that is the Divine.

$\mathcal{F}$IND A PURPOSE

There is a healing power deep within you that can gather and mobilize your life forces to improve your health and extend your life. What is this miraculous healing force? It is the power of purpose—the seventh step in your journey of recovery. Now is the time to find and engage a new purpose for living. With it, a new chapter of your life can begin.

What meaning can anyone's life have if he or she feels no sense of purpose? What would keep a person living, if he or she had no greater motivation than the mere satisfaction of basic appetites? At the core of purpose is love—love of a partner or family member; love of a goal or ambition; love of an endeavor that gives expression to your talents; love as a form of service to your fellow humans, who, like you, have suffered and are in need of help; love of a higher power, which gave you life and placed the will to live inside your very DNA.

The power of purpose was impressively illustrated at the turn of the twenty-first century. On January 15, 2000, the *New York Times* reported that there had been an unusually high death rate in New York City over the first seven days of the year—a death rate far greater than rates seen during the first seven days of previous years. The reason for this dramatic increase in mortalities, scientists speculated, was that the year 2000 held special significance for people. They proposed that those who were close to death and might otherwise have died on or before December 31, 1999, essentially willed themselves to live long enough to see the sun rise on the new millennium.

Richard M. Suzman, associate director of the National Institute on Aging, told the *Times*, "It's pretty well established that people who are seriously ill will hang on to reach significant events, whether they are birthdays, anniversaries, or religious holidays. In this case, making it into the next century or new millennium certainly counts as that." According to Suzman, while the biological mechanisms that prolong life in connection with reaching particular goals are still a mystery, the phenomenon is very real.

Pioneering oncologist Dr. O Carl Simonton noticed this same phenomenon in his treatment of people with cancer. In his book *Getting Well Again*, Dr. Simonton states that, in his experience, those patients who responded well to treatment typically had strong reasons to go on living, though the reasons often varied dramatically. Some wanted to resolve issues with their children or spouses. Others wanted to complete important business transactions. And still others wanted to realize particular ambitions that they had set for themselves. And it shouldn't surprise you too much to know that some of these people made remarkable and unexpected recoveries.

Dr. Simonton recognized early on that the most health-promoting goals were ones that were both highly personal and extremely important to the individual. As he suggests in his book, "Whatever the goals, they had special meaning to the patient—strong enough, apparently, to significantly enhance their will to live." In Dr. Simonton's opinion, "those who are 'around longer' are precisely the ones who make life worth living by investing themselves in something significant to live for."

PEOPLE WITH PURPOSE LIVE LONGER

Since Dr. Simonton made his observations, researchers have conducted numerous studies that have revealed the power of purpose in improving health and extending life. A large experiment done in 2013 by Dr. Patrick Hill and colleagues at Carleton University in Ottawa, Canada, followed more than 6,000 Americans between the ages of twenty-five and seventy for fourteen years. Dr. Hill wanted to know if having a sense of purpose in life could affect longevity.

Among the ways the scientists determined who had purpose and who did not was to probe study participants to discover how they felt about life. People completed psychological questionnaires and were asked if they agreed or disagreed with a series of statements, including the following:

■ Some people wander aimlessly through life, but I am not one of them.

■ I live life one day at a time and don't really think about the future.

■ I sometimes feel as if I've done all there is to do in life.

Dr. Hill and his colleagues found that a greater percentage of people who had a sense of purpose were alive at the end of the study, compared to those who said they were wandering aimlessly or believed they had completed all they had to do in life. Among the more surprising findings was that age was not a significant factor in determining longevity. Young people who felt a sense of purpose lived longer than young people who did not. "Our findings point to the fact that finding a direction for life and setting overarching goals for what you want to achieve can help you actually live longer, regardless of when you find your purpose," explains Dr. Hill in the published report, adding that purpose acts as "a kind of compass or lighthouse that provides an overarching aim and direction to our day-to-day lives."

As cancer researcher Dr. Simonton has pointed out, people can define purpose very differently from one another. One person's purpose may be to provide for his or her family. Another person's may be to live long enough to see a particular milestone—the graduation or marriage of a child, or the arrival of grandchildren. Some people may want to make a significant contribution to society or finish a work of art. "Often individuals want to produce something that is appreciated by others in written or artistic form, whether it's music, dance, or visual arts," says Dr. Hill. For many, purpose can simply be living a healthier life, Dr. Hill also points out.

Your life's purpose should be used as a compass to orient your life, to help you make decisions and engage in behavior that will move you closer to fulfilling that purpose. To be truly meaningful, your purpose should inspire and uplift you toward any goal you wish to accomplish. This inspiration alone can have a healing power.

The Protective Effects of Purpose

Cornell University professor Dr. Anthony Burrow designed a study to discover if merely thinking about one's life's purpose might affect a person's health, especially in reference to a reduction in stress. Dr. Burrow got a group of college student volunteers to ride the Chicago rapid transit system through neighborhoods that were populated by a diverse array of ethnicities and races. Previous research had shown that people experience heightened stress levels—along with all the harmful biological changes that occur in connection with stress—when they are surrounded by groups of people of different ethnicities and races than their own.

Dr. Burrow divided his student volunteers into two groups, each of which rode the same routes through the Chicago transit system. One group of volunteers was instructed to write about a recent movie they had seen.

Each member of the other group wrote about his or her life's direction and purpose. All the student volunteers were given standardized packets, which were used to record their emotional states as they proceeded along the train's path. They were asked to place an X in the box that best described their emotions, as well as the intensity of each emotion, at every stop.

The students who wrote about the last movie they saw experienced significantly heightened stress at each stop, especially when they were surrounded by ethnic and racial groups that were different from their own. The students who each wrote about his or her life's purpose experienced little or no stress at the same stops. Dr. Burrow's study revealed that a sense of purpose protects us against the harmful effects of stress. Perhaps more surprising, however, was the fact that merely thinking about purpose seemed to provide a buffer against stress. As it turns out, other research suggests that the health effects of having a purpose may extend even deeper into human biology—indeed, to our very genes.

Purpose and Biology

Dr. Elizabeth Blackburn, a professor of biochemistry and biophysics at the University of California, San Francisco, won the 2009 Nobel Prize in medicine for her discovery that telomeres, the protective caps on the ends of chromosomes (think of the plastic wrapping around the end of a shoelace), shorten not only with age but also due to chronic stress. As this happens, the chromosomes themselves become vulnerable to fraying. They may also begin to overlap with each other and clump together, causing their genetic information to become chaotic, scrambled, or destroyed. The more this phenomenon occurs, the greater the risk of diseases such as cancer. An enzyme called telomerase slows the erosion of the telomeres, but the body's production of telomerase, too, often declines due to aging and stress.

After she helped discover both telomeres and telomerase, Dr. Blackburn conducted a study in which she placed a group of volunteers in a three-month meditation program to discover what effects meditation might have on their telomeres. She compared the meditation group with a control group that did not meditate. What she found was that the meditation subjects' telomeres actually lengthened, while their telomerase production also increased. This was an important finding, though not entirely surprising, since researchers have long known that meditation can offset the biological effects of stress. What was intriguing was that the meditation subjects experienced an increased sense of purpose in life, which some observers maintained was the real cause of the lengthening of the telomeres and the increased production of telomerase. Those who argued that it was purpose that caused these crucial changes pointed to research showing that purpose alone extends life and improves health, even among people who do not meditate.

Purpose Is Being of Service

Having a sense of purpose often translates into finding ways to help other people in need. And put simply, being of service to another human being is an act of love. In the process, we shift the focus from our own fears and concerns and instead make another person's challenges more important than our own. In the giving of this love, we are momentarily relieved of our own stresses, but more importantly, we are utilizing our own strengths and talents to relieve the pain and suffering of someone else. Somehow, the love we give, the service we render, heals us.

This was the experience of volunteers at Experience Corps, a nonprofit organization that pairs people fifty-five years of age or older with young children who are struggling to develop basic reading and writing skills. The adult volunteers coach students in kindergarten through third grade. Research has shown that the coaching, and perhaps the individual attention, does, indeed, work. The students tend to learn more rapidly and effectively, and both their test scores and morale improve significantly.

When researchers looked at the effects of the coaching on the coaches themselves, they made a remarkable discovery. The adult volunteers experienced significant improvements in several areas of physical, emotional, and mental health. Volunteers saw improvements in mobility, stamina, and flexibility. Those who were depressed when they came to Experience Corp found their depression greatly relieved. At the same time, several improvements in brain function occurred, particularly in memory and decision-making. Confirming the findings at Experience Corp, researchers at Chicago's Rush University found that having a sense of purpose in life was associated with a lower risk of Alzheimer's disease.

It is common belief today to think of caregivers as people who do thankless work and eventually burn out. But one large study published in the *International Journal of Epidemiology* suggests that people who take care of the ill and infirm tend to live longer than those who do not participate in such work. The study, done by researchers at Queen's University in Belfast, Northern Ireland, followed 1.1 million people over thirty-three months. The researchers documented the mortality rates of both caregivers and non-caregivers. Many of the caregivers were indeed overworked, some providing fifty hours or more of service per week. What the researchers found defied expectations. Mortality rates from all causes were far lower in the caregivers than the other participants in the study. Even among caregivers who themselves suffered from physical or emotional problems, the caregivers lived longer than those who were not engaged in similar forms of service. This was true even for the most overworked of the caregivers. For both the men and women who provided fifty hours or more per week, the mortality rate was 27-percent lower for men and 31-percent lower for women compared to non-caregivers.

According to the researchers, "[t]his large population study confirms that for the majority of caregivers the beneficial effects of caregiving . . . appear to outweigh any negative effects, even among people with significant health problems. These results underscore the need for a reappraisal of how caregiving is perceived."

Self-Actualization

As psychologist Abraham Maslow explained, once our most basic needs for survival and safety are met, we naturally turn our attention to our needs for love, belonging, and what he called our greatest need of all, our desire for self-actualization, or the process by which we reach our fullest potentials. Living your purpose is the path toward self-actualization.

One of the remarkable gifts of the healing process is the possibility of self-actualization, which occurs for many as they reach beyond themselves and attempt to help others. The knowledge and wisdom gained from your experience with illness can become the means for you to use your talents to serve the greater good. "We used to call it 'Getting a second bite of the apple,'" says Robert Pritikin, son of the founder of the Pritikin Longevity Center, and the center's former director. For those who have recovered from a seemingly incurable illness, this second chance can be life-changing. As Pritikin suggests, "[m]any of them [want] to do something positive with their lives. They [want] to fulfill a lot of the dreams that they couldn't even think about when they were sick, dreams that they thought had no chance of ever being fulfilled. Every time we get a second chance, we think those kinds of thoughts."

Sometimes "those kinds of thoughts" come from a part of us that is committed to making the world a kinder, gentler place. In Buddhism, this deep desire to be of service, which all of us possess, is called the bodhisattva nature. It is animated by compassion and a desire to bring all sentient beings to a higher state of happiness and awareness. It is common for people who have had a brush with death to awaken to this aspect of our humanity. Having suffered a serious illness, and having been brought to the edge of the abyss, a change comes over each of us. We understand that death is inevitable. It may not come today, but it will come at some point. The knowledge that physical existence has an expiration date awakens us to another dimension of awareness, one that emphasizes spirit over matter, commonalities over differences. In this awareness, compassion, balance, and acceptance of death are guiding principles.

In *The Way of Hope,* I wrote about long-term survivors of AIDS who adopted a healing diet and way of life that led to enhanced immune function and, for some, longer life. Virtually everyone who adopted this way of living recognized its importance to the survival of the gay community at large. Very early in the AIDS crisis, the gay community established an information network to communicate any possible therapies that might be helpful to men suffering from AIDS. The artist Oscar Molini told me what it was like to participate in this network after his healing program had boosted his immune system and extended his life far beyond what his doctors had expected. "I have survived a lot longer than anyone expected, even me," Oscar said in 1985. "If I can go on living and sharing my story with people, my life will have made a difference. I think I've already made a difference. That's very important to me."

Ralph Donsky, about whom I wrote in earlier in this book, also shows us how illness can bring new purpose to life. As his ribs and spinal vertebrae crumbling with every sudden movement, Ralph dreamed about the day when he could use his special talents to be of service to others. Since childhood, Ralph's hobby had been magic tricks, and by the time he had reached adulthood, Ralph was a pretty good magician. As he lay in bed, nearly overcome with despair, Ralph fantasized about performing magic for children and telling people about how he had recovered from a rare form of cancer and a heart attack. "I gave myself the goal of performing magic for children who were ill," Ralph told me. "I spent many hours trying to figure out the best way to present my magic tricks and the stories or patter that would accompany it."

Many people dream about doing such good works one day, but Ralph made good on his promise to himself. After he recovered, he regularly volunteered at St. Francis Medical Center in Hartford, Connecticut, performing his magic show for children and adults with cancer. "The feeling of satisfaction I experienced when I was able to get very ill children to smile or laugh, and to cheer up their families too, was more rewarding than anything I had ever felt in my life," Ralph explained to me. "When I showed my magic to adults, I would add a short inspirational talk about how I had been a patient lying in the same hospital bed, a short time ago. I would bend over to show them the curvature in my upper back and tell them how I almost died from my heart attack and cancer."

Having a purpose is indispensable to recovery. Without purpose, life can seem pointless and futile. We are reduced to being little more than consumers. With purpose, life gains clarity and direction. Your purpose becomes an organizing principle, your guide for making decisions, your reason for being. Purpose gives you the experience of your own uniqueness, as well as your connection to the greater whole, providing the very balance between the personal and the universal that we all seek. In the end, purpose gives you the experience of heroism, which, in turn, can provide you with a sense of connection to the Divine.

ESTABLISHING YOUR HEALING GOALS

People who haven't set goals before becoming ill often find it difficult to articulate exactly what they would like to accomplish besides the overriding goal of getting well. Yet we all need short-term, interim goals to help us achieve our larger ambitions. Goals are the stepping stones to the realization of a purpose for living. Goals can be seen as near-term forms of purpose, which, in turn, lead to your larger purpose.

To enhance your own reflections and help you find your own goals, here are five examples of general goals and the steps that can be taken to achieve them.

My goal is to boost my immune system and recover my health by adopting a healing diet. I will:

- prepare and eat a healing breakfast, lunch, and dinner seven days a week.

- enjoy only healing snacks and desserts. (See Recipes on page 181.)

- avoid all foods that injure my health and impede my healing.

- attend cooking classes to learn how to prepare healing foods and make them delicious and satisfying.

My goal is to improve my health, fitness, energy levels, and endurance. I will:

- walk a specific distance at a specific time of day, six days a week. I will increase this distance by a specific increment every two weeks, or once a month, or to any length I can achieve.

- participate in an additional form of exercise or physical activity that I have always longed to learn, such as a martial art, qi gong, yoga, ballroom dancing, or tennis. I will engage in this new activity one to three times a week.

My goal is to heal my heart, forgive and be forgiven, and bring more love into my life. I will:

- see a loving, supportive, and competent healer or counselor for a specific number of meetings each month.

- attend a support group that is specifically designed to help people who are struggling with challenges similar to my own.

- change a specific pattern or characteristic of my personality that I have identified as an impediment to my happiness and the happiness of those around me.

- recognize and appreciate a specific aspect of my personality (such as humor, wit, humility, compassion, or non-judgment) that makes me happy or makes others happy and find specific ways of expressing that characteristic more often.

- forgive loved ones who have hurt me.

- ask forgiveness of loved ones whom I have injured, and attempt to establish new relationships with loved ones based on forgiveness, compassion, communication, and love.

- spend time and strengthen my relationship with a specific person I love but haven't been with in some time.

- practice expressing my heart, especially to loved ones.

- I will use the Pennebaker method (see page 97) to forgive and heal myself. I will write in a journal at least twice a week to confess all my fears, yearnings, anger, and pain; report my progress on my healing program; express my gratitude; and connect to my inner self and personal needs.

My goal is to improve the quality of my life and to enjoy my life more. I will:

- listen to my body and rest whenever I feel I need to rest, no matter what demands are placed on me.

■ listen to my heart and take a specific amount of time every day to engage in an activity that is meant purely for my own enjoyment, pleasure, or needs.

■ take up a hobby or pastime that I have always wanted to try, such as painting, singing, building model ships, gardening, or learning a second language.

■ carefully plan a visit to a particular place that I have always longed to see, or to a site that has been important in my life.

My goal is to experience or revitalize my spirituality and know myself better. I will:

■ engage in a specific spiritual or religious practice every day.

■ seek out and find an understanding, compassionate, and loving spiritual counselor.

■ practice non-judgment of myself and others and refrain from negative thinking about myself and others.

■ read spiritual or religious literature that uplifts and inspires me a few times a week.

■ find ways to be of service to others through charitable works and by sharing myself in ways that support and express love to others.

■ ask a spiritual or religious group to pray for me. (See Resources on page 217.)

Each of these goals, and the purposes to which they are directed, can have a tremendous impact on your immune system and overall healing power. They are a path to overcoming any illness and restoring your health. Moreover, they are a way back to a healing and loving relationship with the source of all healing.

IDENTIFYING YOUR PURPOSE

The process of identifying and articulating your purpose for living can bring you enormous inner peace and comfort. If you take a little time to reflect, you will discover all kinds of personal desires—both short-term and long-term desires—that have been waiting to be recognized and fulfilled.

Ask yourself, with real compassion, what you would like for yourself right now. Remember what you wanted to become when you were a child. Is any part of that dream relevant to you now? If so, what can you do now to get closer to fulfilling that dream? The answers may be less important than the exercise itself. Sometimes this process can put you in touch with your true nature or your long-denied ambitions.

For many, illness itself can be the stimulus to essential life changes. How many times have we heard of people who, upon being diagnosed with a serious disease, quit the jobs they hated and took up vocations they had always dreamed of pursuing? Your heart may direct you to pastimes that give you pleasure and satisfaction, but which do not appear to the outside world as especially life-changing. How things appear to others is of little or no importance now. The essential step is to listen to your heart and follow its guidance.

One man I know took up pool after being diagnosed with prostate cancer in his late fifties. He had always loved watching the game, but he rarely played it. Now in his late sixties, he is a skilled player and has developed a circle of friends with whom he plays several times a week. He loves the game and it gives him great pleasure every time he plays.

One woman I know resumed her piano lessons after being away from the instrument for more than forty years. "It's the most calming, soothing thing I do," she told me after performing a recital. "It puts me in another world, a very beautiful world." Another man I know committed to learning a second language after meaning to do so for years. He got himself a tutor and studied with her weekly. His goal was to be conversational in this second language, and to travel to a country where he could speak it to the local people.

Your purpose may be no grander than rediscovering a passion or a calling that has lived below the surface of your life without getting the attention you knew it deserved.

Ways to Find Your Purpose

Meditation is one of the most powerful tools available to help you find your purpose. As Dr. Blackburn discovered, regular meditation leads us into deeper recesses of our inner worlds, where the most important answers may be found, including the answer to the question: What should I do with my life? Teachers of meditation ask students to learn to listen to the body. In other words, you should pay attention to how your body reacts when you consider various options that may emerge during meditation. If your body reacts with enthusiasm to a particular idea, pursue this possibility with real passion. If your body reacts as if it has suddenly lost energy, let this idea go. Your body's wisdom is telling you that this path is not for you.

Meditation quiets the mind and allows your soul, your inner knowledge, to guide you to your purpose for living. Follow your meditation with prayer. Promise Spirit that you will stay open to the messages that come to you through your inner voice, from synchronicities and unexpected circumstances, and from messages that may come through friends, family, or people you meet coincidentally. Know that you have a God-given purpose and calling, and that if you open up and listen deeply, you will be led to the opportunities and circumstances where you are most needed.

In addition to meditation, you could write an article or book about your healing journey and put your writings online. Your experience can help many people who find themselves in situations similar to your own. Write your story and share it with the world. Your healing path can be of tremendous service to others. You could also create a website and write an ongoing blog about your life and your recovery experiences, or do a question and answer page where you can answer questions for people seeking alternative and complementary care.

Another way to find your purpose is to create art out of your healing experience. Draw, paint, write a play, or make up a dance. Give artistic expression to your entire journey. If you would like, find a local spot where you could exhibit or perform your artistic creation. Put your work on YouTube or some other online forum.

You could also volunteer your time. Opportunities to volunteer your time, energy, and expertise are virtually endless. Your local community very likely includes many diverse organizations that need experienced people to volunteer their services. Consider counseling or tutoring people in the areas of your expertise. There are numerous volunteer organizations that offer free advice in subjects such as business, law, media, and investing. Look for ways to share the wealth of knowledge you have accumulated over the course of your many years of work and study. The Internet contains a world of volunteer organizations in which you can be of enormous help to people in need. Among these groups is VolunteerMatch.org, which places volunteers in such working areas as animal care, children and youth services, education and literacy, environment, homeless and housing, as well as many other specialty services in cities all across the country. Another useful group, as previously mentioned, is Experience Corps (www.aarp.org/experience-corps), a volunteer organization created by the

AARP. It couples people fifty years or older with kids in kindergarten through third grade in an effort to help these children learn how to read and write.

One of the easiest ways to find your purpose is to read books that might help you discover it. There are many wonderful books that can lead you to your path, including *Find Your Passion* by Derick Van Ness, which leads the reader toward his or her life's purpose by asking questions designed to help the individual rediscover his or her inborn passion. Answer the questions and then meditate on the answers you get. Listen to your inner voice and pray for an opening that would allow you to give expression to the dream that has emerged.

Remember that the answers to your most important questions lie within you, which means they are already present in your life and, more specifically, in that which you love. The challenges you have overcome in your life and the great life lessons you have learned are part of an accumulated wisdom and talent that live within you. But the expression of that talent and wisdom is an act of love and caring. It is this combination of unique life experience, abilities, and love that make you who you are.

Many people have turned extremely challenging and even life-threatening circumstances into great victories and life-long careers. They found their purpose in adversity and went on to live an actualized life by doing what Buddhists call "turning poison into medicine." Nathan Pritikin, as you have read, was just such a man. Pritikin used his illness and all he learned from his recovery to change healthcare in America.

PRITIKIN: THE ACTUALIZED MAN

After he had cured himself of heart disease, Nathan Pritikin began counseling people with serious illnesses, many of whom were beyond medical treatment and in need of miracles. Pritikin treated and healed people using the very methods he had used to heal himself. One such person was Eula Weaver, who, at the age of eighty-one, hobbled into Nathan's office suffering from heart disease, severe angina, high blood pressure, arthritis, and claudication (poor circulation in the legs, which made walking exceedingly difficult). She had already had a heart attack and couldn't walk more than a hundred steps without experiencing severe chest and leg pain. Her circulation was so bad that she had to wear gloves all year round in order to keep her hands warm. After seeing a long list of doctors and taking an array of medications for her numerous conditions, Eula Weaver was diagnosed as beyond hope of recovery—that is, until she met Nathan Pritikin.

Pritikin put her on his diet, taught her to cook whole grains, vegetables, and beans, and asked her not to veer from his recommendations. She didn't. One month later, Pritikin urged Eula to take a short walk each day. Gradually, as her condition improved, he asked her to increase the distance. One year later, Eula was off all medication, free of all her previously severe symptoms, and jogging every day. At the age of eighty-five, Eula entered the Senior Olympics and won two awards, one for the 800-meter race and one for the 1,500-meter race. She competed in the Senior Olympics for six consecutive years, winning twelve awards and becoming a star. Newspapers picked up her story and wrote about this amazing senior athlete who had defied all conventional medical wisdom. This blast of publicity brought Pritikin more patients. He treated them all, with most experiencing tremendous improvements in health. His love of the subjects of diet and health drove him to study their connection further.

In 1975, Pritikin set out to prove that his diet could cure coronary heart disease by conducting an experiment in cooperation with the Veterans Administration Hospital in Long Beach, California. He recruited thirty-eight men, all with proven heart disease. Most of them also suffered from other serious conditions, such a claudication, angina pectoris (chest pain), arthritis, gout, high blood pressure, and high cholesterol levels. He also enlisted Loma Linda University to do angiograms to reveal the degree of atherosclerosis in the men's arteries both before and after the men adopted Pritikin's diet and exercise program.

Six months later, twelve men remained on the program. Their results were better in many respects than Pritikin had dared to hope for. The twelve experienced a 6,000-percent increase in walking distance, the greatest improvement in walking distance in people with claudication ever recorded in the scientific literature. Men who couldn't walk a block at the outset of the study were walking five miles, many ten miles, by the end of the six-month period. All the patients with angina, gout, arthritis, and high cholesterol were relieved of their symptoms and taken off all medication. Of those with high blood pressure, 75 percent of patients saw their readings return to normal and were taken off drugs. One of these men had been on medication for twenty years. Of the group of twelve, two individuals showed reversal of atherosclerosis in the femoral arteries.

Pritikin finished his study and presented its results to the American Congress of Rehabilitation Medicine's national meeting, which was held in Atlanta on November 19, 1975. The next day, the *Atlanta Journal* ran a front page headline that read, "Heart Disease Breakthrough Offers Hope." The

Associated Press picked up the story and it was run in newspapers around the country. In a matter of days, Pritikin was swamped with mail asking for more information on his remarkable program. "And I happened to think," Pritikin would recall years later, "this would be an ideal time to put it into practice. If I wait for the medical community, it will be two hundred years. I better do it myself."

Thus was born the Pritikin Longevity Center, which opened initially in Santa Barbara in 1976 and later moved to Santa Monica and Florida. Since that time, the Longevity Center has treated more than 80,000 people and the results—confirmed repeatedly by independent researchers—have been nothing short of miraculous.

Nathan Pritikin had no college degree and no formal medical education. By conventional standards, he was completely unqualified to have any impact on medicine or healthcare. Yet he saved the lives of thousands. Today, every medically based diet and exercise program is, in one way or another, an extension of his work. He is proof of what can happen when you commit to a life of service and allow the infinite mystery that we refer to as God to determine how your life will unfold. In the meantime, we may take comfort in the words of the Jewish sages, who taught that if you save the life of a single person, you save the entire world.

FROM "ME" TO "WE"

As you begin your healing journey, you must first embrace the need to practice compassion for yourself. This is the foundational principle of recovery, and one that you should never let go. Every step along the healing path is meant to transform you physically, emotionally, and spiritually. As you progress, you will set goals for yourself, goals that will serve as points on a map. Your progress very likely will awaken the part of your humanity that empathizes with the suffering of others, and the fundamental need to be of service. In short, you will go from thinking of yourself as an individual to thinking of yourself as part of a larger whole—less "me," more "we."

Looking back, you will realize that your path has changed you in ways you could not have predicted. You will be stronger, wiser, healthier, and more vibrant. You will have transformed yourself physically, to be sure, but you will also have evolved emotionally, psychologically, and spiritually.

Along your path, you will be guided by mysterious forces. Indeed, your heart and mind will open up to more subtle and sensitive states of being. You will begin to live with a greater intimacy for the tenderness and vulnerability of others and of yourself. You will find yourself capable of greater understanding and love. Your point of view on life will be broader, deeper. Your consciousness will have entered a new realm, a world between Heaven and Earth, where spiritual forces mingle with the temporal and give birth to possibilities that defy rationality, a state of being that we can refer to as the miraculous.

THE HEALING
MIRACLES WITHIN

L ife's challenges have a way of narrowing your focus and reducing your life to fit within the dimensions of your problems. This tendency is especially true if you are battling a serious illness. Under the stress of sickness, you may be tempted to define yourself by the status of your disease, or to think of your body purely in terms of blood values and weight. From there, the lens can narrow even further. Fear can drive you into the false belief that your immune system and healing forces are powerless—perhaps even irrelevant—against your disease, and that only the most aggressive forms of treatment will help you. Thus, you may abandon all forms of complementary care, thinking complementary methods too weak to make a difference. Similarly, fear can cause you to see other people—especially those closest to you—merely as sources of support rather than people who need your love in return.

The fact is that you are more than your disease. Your body is more than any set of numbers that medical science utilizes to define your health. Your loved ones need your caring, which, once you have given it, will benefit you, too. It's essential to remember that your ability to heal flows from a power within you that cannot be seen by x-rays or detected by CT scans, much less understood or appreciated by those who rely exclusively on high-tech diagnostics. Inside of you lies a healing intelligence with powers far beyond the comprehension of anyone's rational faculties. This intelligence has been directing your immune system and healing forces to defeat disease since the day you were born. It is still alive inside you, and in a great many cases its tremendous healing powers can still be brought to bear to restore your health, no matter what your illness may be.

The real work of healing is to align your focus, faith, and most of all your actions with this healing power. This does not mean abandoning medical treatment. On the contrary, medical treatment can often help you align with your healing intelligence. But in the end, all true and lasting healing lies with a power already present in your life. Let's examine this awesome force and learn how you can align your life with it in order to draw upon its miraculous powers.

THE MAESTRO MANAGING
THE UNIVERSE WITHIN

Your body is made of about 100 trillion cells, more cells by far than there are stars in the Milky Way. Each of your cells is doing its own highly differentiated job—those that make up your brain are helping you think; those in your eyes are helping you see; those in your gut are helping you digest food and eliminate waste; those in your heart are helping pump blood more than 100,000 times a day. Even as your cells do their jobs, they are constantly communicating with each other to ensure that they are in harmony with the whole of your body.

Within each of your cells is your DNA, or genome, which is made of up more than 20,000 genes. These genes produce proteins that serve as blueprints—or instructions—for the mass production of proteins throughout your body, some of which serve as building blocks for your physical body, some of which act as messengers that direct cells to function properly, and some of which make it possible for cells to communicate with each other.

One can hardly think about such a massive orchestration of cellular and genetic activity without wondering how it is possible to manage 100 trillion cells, make precise genetic decisions, and ensure that every cell functions for the good of the whole organism. The answer is summed up in a single word: information. Countless trillions of commands are communicated from an incomprehensible intelligence to every cell in your body at every instant of every day. Exactly how this information is transmitted to these cells is a mystery for which no human being truly has an answer. Only the maestro that conducts this 100-trillion-instrument symphony knows how this feat is accomplished. But researchers are starting to understand some of the events that take place within this seemingly incomprehensible communications network.

Inside each cell are tiny chemical messengers called kinases, which speed along pathways at breathtaking speeds—faster than 100 meters per second. These kinases travel to precise points on the genome in order to throw certain switches—turning on some genes and turning off others, depending on the orders from the maestro. This job is even more complicated than it sounds, as kinases need to make their way through a labyrinth of convoluted twists and turns.

Some time ago, I spent an afternoon with Dr. James Broach, who at the time was the associate director of the Lewis-Sigler Institute for Integrative Genomics at Princeton University. (Today he is chair of the department of biochemistry and molecular biology at Penn State and the director of the Penn State Institute for Personalized Medicine.) In order to help me understand (even a little) how truly daunting the job of intracellular communication is, Dr. Broach pulled out a scientific journal and pointed to a schematic that documented a cell's inner network of pathways. It looked like a map of the Southern California highway system, only doubled.

Along these pathways, each kinase must make intricate turns in order to find exactly the right gene to activate or deactivate. No one knows how the body's intelligence guides a tiny protein along the cellular equivalent of the Los Angeles freeway system to an exact location on the genome, but it does. As you might expect, there is a lot at stake. "The decisions a cell makes determines whether you maintain health or whether your body is thrown off homeostasis, such as when you suffer from a disease such as diabetes," Dr. Broach told me. This means that these tiny proteins within 100 trillion cells better get it right.

As if all of this were not complicated enough, consider that cells are receiving a continual stream of information from all over your body, such as your blood levels of oxygen, glucose, insulin, essential proteins, and disease-causing agents, as well as the relative state of your immune support, just to name a handful of data points. Each cell has to make sense of all this information and then immediately react to create the right genetic sequences so that you function coherently, and, of course, go on living.

Cellular communication occurs not just within cells but also between them. Cells are organized in neighborhoods. Like billions of synchronized swimmers, the cells in these neighborhoods have to perform in exact harmony in order for organs, systems, and senses to function properly. This task gets even more challenging when you consider that the swimmers have to juggle hundreds, if not thousands, of bits of data while they swim in unison. Picture every Chinese citizen doing advanced synchronized swimming in perfect unison while each one juggles several hand grenades. Maybe this image gets us a little closer to understanding the reality occurring inside of each of us. Cells manage this feat by being in a state constant communication with the overriding intelligence and with each other, which they manage to do through the crisscrossing of another set of protein signals called cytokines.

"For many years, we as biologists have been studying how any one signal impinges on and changes the behavior of a cell," said Dr. Broach. "And we have learned that different signals change the cell in different ways. Some signals tell the cell to grow, some tell it to stop growing. What we are learning now is that the cell doesn't get a single signal, but multiple signals at the same time, and it has to decide what is the appropriate response at that moment." And they do so with a beauty, grace, and perfection that inspires both awe and reverence. Anyone who has, so to speak, looked under the hood of the human body cannot help but marvel at this wonder of wonders. Health is a gift from an intelligence that can never be matched in genius, precision, or effectiveness by any array of drugs, surgical procedures, or technological advances known to humankind. In fact, when we consider the remarkable recovery stories described in this book, a single blinding insight emerges: Something lives inside of us that is superior to all forms of illness. Indeed, it has been conquering illness every day, in every human being, since the dawn of human life on the planet. But, of course, our recognition of this intelligence begs a series of challenging questions: How is it that this marvelous power is ever thwarted? How can such a beautiful harmony go wrong? And since we are busy asking questions, we might as well ask the ultimate one, which is: When that which makes us tick is disabled or crashes, can we reboot and make it right again? If so, then how?

The short answer to the first two questions is simple. All too often, we get in the way. Our diets, sedentary lifestyles, thinking patterns, emotional states, stress levels, and behaviors—in short, the results of modern life—create chaos within the system and thus disrupt the delicate communication between the maestro and the living universe that each of us really is. How do we restore the harmony? We restore the lines of communication between the maestro and our cells. How do we do this? We must live in alignment with the intelligence that is directing the unfathomable symphony. The seven steps described in this book will help you accomplish this goal.

THE MAESTRO AND ITS NATURE

Among the most important keys to restoring communication between the intelligence and your cells is to restore order within your system. This means, in effect, to restore biochemical balance and reduce biological chaos.

When this happens, healing miracles are indeed possible, simply because the healing intelligence within you is capable of overcoming even the most advanced illness.

Restoring communication within your system is actually not as difficult as it sounds. Each of the seven steps in this book has a profound effect on health, partly because each does exactly that—it restores biological balance and reduces the chaos. I would like to show you how each step moves you along the path of reestablishing healthful communication between your cells and the healing intelligence living inside you.

Get Past the Shock

Fear can make it exceedingly difficult, and sometimes impossible, for your cells to receive the commands from the healing intelligence. The steps described in this book can take you out of fear and create stability for your cells and overall body and mind. This stability will allow your cells to receive the commands from the healing intelligence and form the basis for healing miracles.

Fear and what is euphemistically referred to as chronic stress produce high levels of dopamine, norepinephrine, adrenaline, and a cascade of stress hormones, collectively referred to as catecholamines. When elevated beyond certain levels, these chemicals cause body-wide physical tension, biological chaos, and even more fear, all of which can have destructive effects on the heart, circulation, respiration, digestion, and kidney function.

What many people fail to consider are the energetic consequences of fear—in other words, fear's effects on the vibration of cells. Every cell in your body oscillates, and under healthy conditions, cells vibrate at their own frequency ranges. When vibrating within these healthy ranges, cells can easily receive instructions from the intelligence that governs their activities. But once they start oscillating at higher frequencies that are outside their comfort zones, these chaotic oscillations drive biochemical processes that are themselves highly destructive to health.

As you know, whenever you are afraid, your body may literally tremble. The reason for this reaction is simple: Fear generates intense electromagnetic waves that start in your brain and travel throughout your body. These waves, referred to as high beta waves, vibrate within frequency ranges of 22 to 50 cycles per second, or cps. And at these intense frequencies, every cell in your body is affected. Various kinds of diagnostic tests—including electroencephalographs (EEG), electrocardiograms (EKG), and even polygraph tests—produce tracings of the various frequency states we may experience. Anyone who has ever seen tracings of high beta waves knows that they are characterized by extremely high peaks and valleys, meaning the waves reach high above and well below the median line. High beta frequencies are big waves, chaotic, highly unstable, and extremely powerful.

As long as cells continue to vibrate within high beta ranges, they cannot receive the more subtle communication from the healing intelligence. In the process, they fall out of alignment with the intelligence that would restore the body to health.

Every step described in this book is capable of defeating fear and the biochemical chaos it creates. Each step creates a deeper sense of peace, balance, and relaxation. It does so by tamping down the biological noise created by fear and stress, replacing it with states of relative interior silence, which allow cells to listen again to their true master. This is merely the first step in restoring communication with the healing intelligence within you.

Take Back Your Power

When it comes to health and healing, power comes from the willingness to make your own health decisions. It arises from the knowing that healing, ultimately, is a solitary path. You must listen to all the experts and their counsel. But in the end, you, in deep connection with the healing intelligence within you, must be the one who decides the path you will travel.

Giving up your power has a disintegrating effect on your psyche, especially when you are plunged into a health crisis. A cacophony of voices may pull your thoughts in all directions. You may wonder, *Whom should I listen to? Whom can I trust? What should I do?* Powerlessness can also lead to a form of anger that turns inwardly on itself and outwardly on innocent people who are trying to help. Like fear, anger charges the brain with high beta waves—high amplitude, intense, and chaotic—which cut off communication with the guiding intelligence within.

Powerless anger often leads to depression, and then to deeper states of fear and confusion. In such a state, people all too often surrender their wills to authority figures who may present an air of power and knowledge, but who may not have anything to offer of any real therapeutic value. Taking back your power and making your own decisions has a coalescing effect on your psyche. It creates greater integration and stability. It brings you out of the chaotic high beta cycles and into what is referred to as mid to low beta states. Mid beta frequencies range from 16 to 22 cycles per second; low beta from 13 to 15 cps. In a mid beta state, you have the ability to put information together in a coherent picture, analyze the data, and think a problem through. Stress levels are far lower than they are in high beta states. Low beta states are experienced when, for example, you are reading a book or having a relaxed conversation with another person. These are low stress states.

At these lower frequencies, you naturally experience a greater sense of peace, better rest, and enhanced clarity of thought. You feel time slow down. You can consider your options in a more open, intelligent state of mind. All of these body-wide symptoms are the consequences of an inner peace at the cellular level. Your cells are vibrating at frequencies that are closer to their natural states. And at these ranges, they are more likely to be guided by the healing intelligence that can give you the experience of knowing the right decision for your own body at any given moment.

Taking back your power also restores your conscious connection to the warrior archetype, which is the carrier of your courage and stability, and your conscious connection to your truth. The warrior is willing to walk his or her own path—a path based on one's own deep knowledge and inner conviction. Yes, the warrior takes in information from all sources—medical and complementary—and makes its own decisions based on an inner knowledge that flows from the healing intelligence within.

Before you make any health decision, take time to feel what you believe to be right and true for you. Take walks. Be in nature. Eat simply. Sit in the sun. Watch the rain. Reach deeply into your inner self. Meditate. Pray. Be in sacred places—a church, synagogue, or temple. Step out of fear and feel what the inner intelligence is guiding you to do. As you gain emotional stability, you will experience a greater capacity to listen to the healer within, and to know intuitively the right decision for you.

Adopt a Healing Diet

Plant foods eliminate extremes in your biochemistry. In other words, they restore balance and harmony to your system, and boost the ability of your cells to receive the restorative commands of the healer within.

When we consider the three driving forces behind common degenerative conditions—high insulin, high inflammation, and obesity—we are actually looking at biochemical overstimulation. In a word, chaos, which means that on the typical modern diet, effective communication between your cells and the healing intelligence within you is virtually impossible. As previously described, insulin is a powerful mitogen, which is a chemical substance that commands cells to divide and multiply. In this way, it stimulates cell growth beyond what is needed for the body to function in an orderly, controlled, and healthy way. Insulin is highly stimulating. Cancer, an illness associated with an overproduction of cells, needs insulin to stimulate rapid, uncontrolled cell growth, and thus requires insulin in order to thrive.

When insulin levels are high, so are glucose levels. This means that your cells have to work extra hard to burn off as much of the excess glucose and insulin as they can. In most cases, cells can burn off only a fraction of the excess fuel. Whatever remains gets stored as body fat, which, of course contributes to rapid and escalating weight gain. Remarkably, even storing the excess fuel will not reduce the entire glucose load, and eventually both the excess glucose and insulin will make your cells insulin resistant, a disorder that leads to a multitude of disease states, as previously described.

Inflammation is essentially war within your arteries, tissues, and organs. It is the immune system battling for your life. And as the battle rages, tremendous collateral damage is done. Many healthy cells die, while others mutate and become diseased. Fat cells become factories for highly inflammatory compounds, among them estrogen, a hormone that acts like both insulin and growth factors, telling cells to divide and multiply. Estrogen grows tissue and blocks circulation of lymph and blood in many sensitive areas of the body, including the breast and reproductive organs. When insulin, inflammation, and weight are all high, you are, in essence, flogging your cells to work themselves sick. The vibratory state of your cells is pure chaos. Under such conditions, cells become overstimulated. Cellular function becomes so disorderly that many cells simply die, while others become scar tissue, and still others mutate and become malignant.

A plant-based diet changes these conditions for the better. It cools the body and takes it out of acute inflammatory states, thus reducing and, in many cases, eliminating inflammation's detrimental effects. It restores insulin to normal, healthy ranges, and thus releases the body from a state of overstimulation. It can dramatically lower weight and reverse the activities of fat cells—converting them from toxin-producers into makers of healing compounds, including adiponectin, a powerful health-producing protein.

A plant-based diet strengthens the immune system and positively transforms the internal environment, eliminating many of the poisons that sicken organs and tissues throughout the body. Looking deep within the cell itself, we see that plant food even changes the way genes function, altering them so dramatically that they no longer create the genetic conditions for sickness but rather for health. In other words, it helps genes receive commands from the internal intelligence that is capable of restoring health.

Create a Supportive Community

Love is the giving of energy that nourishes and supports life. Love's very essence is energy, meaning a specific and very powerful set of waves that transform the body and take it out of the high beta frequencies, causing the entire body to relax, open up, and receive even more love (in the form of energy) from the outer environment and, most importantly for those battling illness, from the healer within.

The steps described in this book can improve your health in many ways, but among the most powerful is by transforming the wave patterns that currently dominate your body. Among the most powerful ways you can do this is to establish a healing community and work with a team of healers.

You will recall Dr. Elmer Green, the physicist introduced in step four, who measured the amount of energy given off by highly adept healers. Dr. Green found that some healers could transmit enormous quantities of energy, in some cases 190 volts, which amounts to 100,000 times the normal energy output produced by the human body.

Healers who are truly effective at channeling abundant flows of healing energy will tell you that as they do their work, they concentrate on compassion, a form of love. Compassion facilitates the flow of healing energy. The healing intelligence within communicates its commands via this same energy, which is love. As you have been shown throughout this book, love heals. No matter whether we are talking about healing touch, the love of an intimate partner, the love in someone's voice and words, the love of family, the positive beliefs that support placebo (also a form of love), the love in the food you eat, or the gentle and loving way you take care of your body, all of these are simply different manifestations of the same energetic force, which we call love.

Boost the love in your life—in as many ways as you can—and the healer within will be able to do the rest.

Commit to Healing

Commitment to healing is solidified when you adopt healing behaviors and follow them consistently. Among the most powerful tools for strengthening your commitment is rhythmic exercise, which is itself a series of gentle wave patterns that are in alignment with your energy level, the needs of your body, and the healer within.

To commit means to focus. It means to put certain values, behaviors, and people at the top of your priority list. You are defined by your commitments. Why? Because your commitments require more of your time and energy, which means they require more of your life. In a practical, experiential way, commitment really means starving a certain part of you—the part that, in the past, was engaged in certain ways of thinking, eating, and behaving, which, in their own ways, diminished your body's capacity to receive the guidance of the healer within. Commitment also means nourishing and growing another part of you that you are now becoming— the person who lives in alignment with the healing intelligence within you. This new version of you confronts your fears and overcomes them. It listens to your health advisors but makes its own health decisions. It eats a plant-based diet and avoids all processed food, sugar, and high-fat animal products. It is engaged in loving activities with loving family, friends, and healers. It is committed to living a new way of life, a way of life that is grounded in the healing behaviors described in this book. It is committed to creating a life that is based on listening to the "still, small voice within," and the gentle impulse that arises within your body whenever you suddenly experience your own truth, your own deep knowledge that this is the path you should follow. This impulse is a message full of inspiration and information, flowing from the healing intelligence inside of you.

Among the best ways to focus is through rhythmic exercise practiced gently, consciously, and regularly. Good examples of this are walking, gentle stretching, yoga, rhythmic movement such as dancing, and rhythmic martial arts such as qi gong or tai chi chuan. Exercise done in rhythm, as described in step five, connects you to your own inner life, where the healing intelligence can be found constantly communicating healing instructions to your every cell.

Rhythmic exercise can be a form of meditation. As you feel the flow of the movement, your mind can stop its train of thought, which is one of the principal sources of chaotic energy. Instead, you can bring your awareness to your body and inner life and experience the peace and harmony that arises when you are in alignment with your inner healer.

During exercise, try to listen to your body as it tells you when you have the energy and strength to speed up, when to exert yourself a little more, when to slow down, and when to rest. Trust your body's signals. It is transmitting to your awareness the information it receives from the healing intelligence within. Remember, there is a healing genius inside you, guiding your way back to health. Commitment means learning to listen to it. No longer should your mantra be "No pain, no gain." Now you must say to yourself, *Trust the Inner Intelligence, have faith in the healer within.*

Believe in Your Ability to Heal

Prayer and meditation are the two sides of a healing conversation with your Creator. Prayer is you speaking to the Creator. Meditation is you listening in silence to the Infinite's flow of information, which proceeds through the awesome intelligence within you and manifests as the "still, small voice within" through the "still, small impulse" that flares in your body when you know that something is true or right for you, and through the countless synchronicities that are experienced on your healing journey.

Belief is essential, especially in the early stages of your healing journey. You must believe in the good within yourself, in the good in others, in the good within the medical treatments you decide to utilize, and the good in your complementary healing methods. Without belief, your own innate healing powers will retreat from the treatments you utilize and thus will weaken these treatments or render them powerless against your illness.

On the other hand, eventually belief has to square with the reality of your experience. It must correspond to what is true for you in your body, heart, mind, and soul. It must be true in your daily life. When your beliefs rest on the bedrock of your experience and a more intimate connection with the inner intelligence that is guiding your recovery, then your beliefs are transformed into faith. Faith arises when you start to see the effects of the inner healer in your life and you begin to realize, on the basis of these small successes, where your efforts are leading. You realize that you are living more and more in alignment with the inner intelligence. You feel yourself changing for the better.

For example, let's say that you adopt a plant-based, healing diet, and in a matter of a few weeks or a couple of months, you experience a healing response from within your body. You have more energy; you sleep more deeply and more restfully; you feel a greater sense of well-being. You realize that your approach is working. You feel your body getting stronger. In time, you realize that the underlying transformation is gaining momentum.

This example could be applied to every one of the steps in this book. You start out believing that perhaps each step could have a healing effect on your condition. But then you fully engage in each step and experience their effects. You realize that your feelings about your recovery are no longer based exclusively on belief but also on your experience. There may not be enough information to know the outcome yet, but you are starting to experience faith in the process and where it is leading. You realize that the big prayer is being answered, that the big miracle is possible. Meditation is a key to this process because meditation is the act of clearing your mind of all the dissonant energies that encumber the healing intelligence from communicating its messages effectively to your cells.

In meditation, your goal is to quiet your mind so that you can be free of the fear-and confusion-producing beta cycles. As your mind relaxes and its thoughts are allowed to drift away, your brain settles into an alpha state, which refers to brain frequencies between 8 and 13 cycles per second. At these frequencies, the mind is quiet and finds rest, and your body experiences healing.

As you meditate, observe your mind without being pulled into any thought, feeling, or emotional drama that your brain may conjure up as a way to pull you into chaos. Simply observe your thoughts and let them go. Witness the parade of images and feelings without interest as they pass through your awareness and disappear into oblivion. In this silence and stillness are your answers. Without chatter, confusion, and fear occupying your mind, your healing intelligence can communicate effectively with your body. This is how all the good occurs.

It doesn't matter if you do not hear that still, small voice, or feel any sudden impulse within your body. Simply hold the silence so that the healing intelligence and your cells can do their good work. At this point, miracles are possible.

Find a Purpose

Sooner or later, the vast majority of us come to realize that our actions are meaningful only insofar as they are expressions of love. In the end, we see that only love can create that which all of us are seeking—health, fulfillment, joy, and peace. At the core of all the commands issued by the healing intelligence is this energy—the very distinct and powerful waves that are love. Why is this true? Because love is the one and only force on earth that can unify opposites. It is the singular force that can restore communication and health between conflicting cells, organs, and people. This is what the healing intelligence seeks to do every instant of every day that you are alive in a physical body.

When we consider the intelligence that is orchestrating your recovery, we come face to face with a genius of infinite proportion whose singular mission is to keep you healthy and alive in a physical body for as long as possible. Why this is so is a mystery no one is going to solve. What we can know, however, is the joy and satisfaction we all experience when we help another human being.

The healing intelligence seeks to help you. Given the right conditions, it can orchestrate a cellular harmony that may restore your health. Once this is accomplished, this intelligence can—through so many improbable coincidences—create situations in which you can be of service to others. As you become engaged in this service, it rewards you with feelings of deep satisfaction and joy. Thus its nature is revealed. In this way, your life takes on great meaning and significance. Indeed, being of service may be the penultimate step on the healing journey, because your work is no longer just about you, but about all of us. In this way, you, and the awesome intelligence within you, are fulfilled.

THE NORMAN ARNOLD STORY

In 1982, Norman Arnold, then fifty-two, was one of the most successful men in all of South Carolina. Married and the father of three sons, Norman had only recently sold his wine and spirits distribution company, the Ben Arnold Company, after making it the largest such retail company in the state, and among the top ten in the country. Having achieved all the financial success he could have dreamed of, he was now looking around for something to do with the rest of life, something that gave his life purpose, meaning, and even rebirth. So far, nothing had shown up.

Norman had one small physical problem, however: he had a nagging pain in his back that had persisted for nearly a year. His doctors weren't sure what was wrong, but most agreed that it must be his gallbladder. On July 27, 1982, he entered Providence Hospital in Columbia, South Carolina, and was operated on the following day. The surgery was expected to be routine. It was anything but.

The surgeon who performed the operation was a long-time friend of Norman's, Dr. Dan Davis. Dr. Davis opened Norman's abdomen and was about to turn his attention to Norman's gallbladder when he decided to examine the other organs that were now available for inspection. He scrutinized Norman's pancreas and discovered a tumor the size of an egg. He also found what he suspected were three cancerous lesions on Norman's liver. Dr. Davis biopsied the pancreatic tumor and the three lesions and sent the samples to pathology for analysis. He then turned his attention to Norman's gallbladder and, as expected, found that it was filled with gallstones. He removed the organ, closed the abdominal incision, and sent Norman to intensive care.

Because Norman was an important patient—a hospital donor and well-known throughout the community—his pathology report came back within hours. Its conclusion was unequivocal: The pancreatic tumor and all three liver lesions were malignant.

Pancreatic cancer is incurable, with an average life expectancy of about five months after diagnosis. After learning the pathology report results, Dan Davis went to the waiting room and found Norman's wife, Gerry Sue. He escorted her to the lounge and proceeded to tell her, as gently as he could, how perilous Norman's condition was.

"It took time for his words to register," Gerry Sue recalled. "I kept asking him what we would do next and he gently explained that there really wasn't anything left to do." Two terrifying questions kept pressing themselves into her mind, but Gerry Sue dared not ask them: *Is Norman going to die? If so, how much time does he have to live?* But she had to know.

"We have reservations for a skiing trip at Christmas, Dan," Gerry Sue said obliquely. "Can Norman go on that trip?"

"I think you should go," Dr. Davis said.

Gerry Sue's mind raced. "We've got a bar mitzvah in April. What about that?"

Dr. Davis paused, calculating the months. "Can you move it up?" he asked.

Gerry Sue had her answer.

When Norman was awake, Dr. Davis came into the ICU, sat down on the end of his bed, and gave his friend the terrible news: Norman had adenocarcionoma of the pancreas with metastatic lesions to the liver. The situation was hopeless. Norman could expect to live perhaps five to nine months, tops. Once he had told Norman the news, Dr. Davis left the room and Gerry Sue rushed in. The two embraced and, as he would say much later, Norman felt the world collapse around him. "We're all sitting ducks," he muttered.

Norman was soon moved to a private room, where an oncologist, Dr. Bill Babcock, explained that Norman should undergo chemotherapy. Norman questioned the effectiveness of such a procedure on his illness. The chemotherapy would have only a marginal effect, Dr. Babcock admitted.

"As I listened to his words, I disengaged from reality," Norman recalled. "I sank into my pillow and entered a fog."

When Dr. Babcock left, Gerry Sue tried to assure Norman that the two of them would fight this disease. "Our first few conversations were us grasping at empty hope," Norman recalled. "We were just fighting the darkness."

Later, Norman forced himself to think about his situation and what he could do. "I still had my three sons to raise," he told himself. "My wife was still young. Since I was an only child, my mother would be left without her son to care for her. But there was also an emptiness in my soul. I had been given a great deal by life, but I had the sense that I had not given back all that I should have. And now everything was about to be washed away."

At this point, Norman was in despair. He realized that he had reached the limits of what conventional medicine could give him. Yes, there were possible experimental treatments out there, but they were long shots at best. He knew that if he became a compliant patient, and surrendered to his doctors, he would soon be dead. He had to regain his composure and somehow take control of his situation. The first thing he decided was to get out of the hospital. Nothing positive could be done from his bed; and lying there only made him feel like a victim.

On the afternoon of August 5, 1982, Gerry Sue arrived at Providence Hospital and proceeded to make her way to Norman's room. She had regained her characteristic composure and, like Norman, was ready to find something—anything—that might help her husband. When she entered Norman's room, she was shocked to find him dressed and ready to bolt. Even before she had a chance to say hello, Norman announced, "I'm getting out of here. Either you're going to drive me or I'm calling a cab." With that, he marched down the hallway of the hospital and headed for the door. A nurse ran after him like a chicken announcing the presence of a fox.

"Mr. Arnold, Mr. Arnold, you can't leave, you can't leave, sir," she said.

"My dear, I am doing just that," Norman replied and didn't lose a step.

"You can't do that, Mr. Arnold. You'll have to sign some papers before we can let you go," she said. "The hospital can't take responsibility for you if you leave now, sir."

"That's fine," said Norman. "Where do I sign?"

It took a few minutes to gather the paperwork and, without even reading it, Norman signed his name and headed for the parking lot, Gerry Sue hurrying at his elbow. He was only a few feet inside his front door when the phone rang. Dr. Davis was on the other end.

"Norman, you left before I had a chance to take out your stitches," he said. Norman had been in such a hurry to leave that he didn't consider the sutures or the small tube in his side that was meant to allow fluid and air to drain from his abdomen. This, too, would have to be removed.

"That's right, Dan," said Norman. "When do you want to take them out?"

"I'm leaving for the beach tonight. I'll be over this evening." That night, Dr. Davis arrived at Norman's house. He had Norman lie on his kitchen table where he plucked the stitches from his body and closed off the drain.

"I felt like a big bird being prepared for the oven," said Norman. "But at least I felt some control over my life again."

With the help of his cousin, Dr. Charles Banov, Norman immediately began considering the possible treatment options that were available to him. Standard chemotherapy was out of the question, since the evidence clearly showed that it was useless against his illness. All the other treatment options were experimental. One of them was malaria therapy, which involved injecting the cancer-afflicted organ with malaria in the hope that the resulting fever might kill the cancer. Another, hyperthermia treatment, treated the cancerous organ by heating the organ in the hope that the heat would also kill the cancer. Neither of these seemed to offer much promise.

Two other experimental treatments seemed vaguely plausible. One was an experimental chemotherapy, which might extend Norman's life by one year. The drugs, which would have severe side effects, would be administered as part of a larger study done at Georgetown Medical Center in Washington, D.C. The other experimental approach was monoclonal antibodies, which were antibodies produced by mice that had been injected with human blood containing cancer. It was theorized that the mouse would produce antibodies against the cancer. These antibodies would be removed from the mouse and injected into the patient where, it was hoped, they would help the patient's body overcome the cancer. Among the ways the mouse antibodies would do that is by stimulating the patient's own immune system to produce similar antibodies that would be effective at killing the cancer. There was no proof that the monoclonal antibodies might work against pancreatic cancer, or any other type, but the idea appealed to Norman.

Norman decided to pursue both experimental treatments.

But then the unexpected happened. Without being asked, another of Norman's cousins, Sandy Gottlieb, arrived one day with the current issue of *Life* magazine. It featured an article about a Dr. Anthony Sattilaro, who had used a macrobiotic diet to recover from his own terminal cancer. Dr. Sattilaro had been diagnosed with prostate cancer that had spread throughout his body. After much unsuccessful surgery and hormone therapy, Dr. Sattilaro was given between eighteen months and three years to live. A short time later, he adopted the macrobiotic diet. Within eighteen months, bone tests, x-rays, and blood analyses revealed no sign of his cancer. The magazine published before-and-after photographs of Dr. Sattilaro's bone scans, illustrating the presence of cancer before the diet, and the absence of malignancy a year and a half later.

"Had I not been ill, the macrobiotic diet would not have appealed to me in the slightest," Norman recalled, "but given the desperation of my circumstances I now thought seriously of looking into it. I placed macrobiotics at the very top of my list."

Norman wanted to meet people in South Carolina who practiced macrobiotics. He called the Kushi Institute, the Boston-area macrobiotic teaching center mentioned in *Life* magazine. A person there gave him the name of Becky Kabuto, a macrobiotic cook who lived in Asheville, North Carolina. Norman called Becky and asked if she could teach him and Gerry Sue the basics of the macrobiotic diet. Becky and her Japanese husband arrived at Norman's house the following day.

Becky was in her mid-twenties. She was shy and sweet and six months pregnant. Becky and her husband, who spoke little English, brought a variety of macrobiotic staples, including brown rice, vegetables, a salad press, and several kinds of seaweed. They established themselves in Gerry Sue's kitchen and proceeded to cook a meal. As they did, Becky instructed Gerry Sue and Norman on macrobiotic cooking and philosophy.

The basic idea was that Norman's previous diet and lifestyle was the cause of his cancer. His former diet—rich in fat, sugar, and chemical additives—had caused the accumulation of toxins within his system. These toxins, Becky told them, affected the DNA of his cells and caused the onset of cancer. The macrobiotic diet would help rid his body of the illness by eliminating the toxins that were supporting the life of the cancer. As Becky explained, the whole philosophy of macrobiotics revolved around the idea of balance.

Becky was no scientist or doctor, but she was so sincere and so obviously altruistic in her motivation that Norman could not help but be moved. Her simple and unpretentious explanation of how diet worked had a sort of poetic persuasiveness to it, Norman thought. In addition, she gave him a gem of an image that would prove reassuring later on. Becky said that once Norman's blood became healthy, it would erode the tumors in his body. The cancer would melt away, she said. Norman liked that image a lot.

After preparing the meal, Becky and her husband left the Arnold house. Gerry Sue, Norman, and their three sons ate their first macrobiotic meal. Their dinner that night consisted of brown rice, a variety of green vegetables, a seaweed called hijiki, and navy beans. "The meal wasn't bad," Norman decided. Moreover, the philosophy behind the diet fascinated him. He had always been vaguely interested in nutrition, but his past orientation was toward vitamins and vitamin therapy. But the idea that diet was the foundation of health sounded right to him. Still, he needed more.

On August 9, 1982, Norman went in for another CT scan in an attempt to confirm or deny the earlier diagnosis. The CT scan confirmed the presence of tumors on Norman's pancreas and liver. On August 11, Gerry Sue, Dr. Charles Banov, and Norman went to Georgetown University to meet Dr. Phillip Schein, one of the world's preeminent specialists on pancreatic cancer, and the man who was conducting the study on experimental chemotherapy for pancreatic cancer. Dr. Schein was an impressive man who radiated competence and professionalism. Yet he gave Norman little hope. Dr. Schein knew better than anyone in the world that Norman faced a death sentence. Instead of offering a cure, Dr. Schein offered the possibility of time.

"How long will the chemotherapy give me?" Norman asked.

"Some patients survive eighteen months on this protocol," Dr. Schein said. He pointed out that new therapies were being discovered and that within eighteen months a new method of treatment might be available.

Gerry Sue and Norman were buoyed by the possibility that he might survive a year and a half. They were grateful for that small hope. Norman agreed to undergo the treatment, but only if he had Dr. Schein's assurance that he would be his patient first, and a member of his study second. "Dr. Schein, I need you to assure me that as your patient I will take precedence over your study," Norman said. Norman also wanted to feel confident that Dr. Schein would tell him the truth if, at any point in his treatment, the chemotherapy appeared to be doing him more harm than good. Dr. Schein assured him that he would. Norman agreed to return to Georgetown on August 17 for his first round of chemotherapy. The remainder of the first treatment series would be administered at his primary hospital by his oncologist, Dr. Bill Babcock.

As Norman pursued the two experimental treatments, his mind kept coming back to macrobiotics. He went to a local bookstore and asked for anything the clerk had on macrobiotics. There were a couple of books, including one by Jean Kohler, who, remarkably, had used macrobiotics to help himself recover from pancreatic cancer. The book was entitled *Healing Miracles from Macrobiotics*. Norman bought the book, and he and Gerry Sue read it from cover to cover that night.

Another round of telephone calls yielded the telephone number of Michio Kushi, the leading teacher of macrobiotics. When he called Kushi's home in Brookline, Massachusetts, a secretary answered. Norman explained the reason for his call. It would be impossible for him to see Michio Kushi, the secretary told Norman, because Kushi was leaving for Europe that evening. He'd be gone for about a month.

"Does he have any time to see me this afternoon?" Norman asked.

"Yes," she said. "He could see you at 5 PM for about an hour."

"Well, I'll be there at 5 PM today. I'll be traveling from Columbia, South Carolina, so you won't be able to get back in touch with me to cancel," I said.

She asked Norman his name and told him that Mr. Kushi would see him at 5 PM. As soon as Norman hung up the phone, he called the Columbia airport and charted the next available plane for Boston. A few hours, Norman and Gerry Sue landed at Logan Airport in Boston, and took a cab to the Kushi house in Brookline. The house was an enormous stone mansion with a large portico before the front door. "It reminded me of the television show *The Munsters,*" Norman recalled. "I didn't know what to make of the place."

Soon they were ushered into a large library that was solid with books. Michio Kushi got up from a chair and hurried over to them with his secretary a step behind. The minute Norman saw Michio, he had a good feeling. He was smiling and greeting them in an unpretentious, warm-spirited way. The three shook hands and Michio directed Gerry Sue and Norman to a small alcove off the library that had large windows through which the late afternoon light entered. Once the three were seated, Norman told Michio the full extent of his illness and the options that he faced. Kushi listened carefully and then proceeded to give Norman a very strange examination, looking closely at his face, eyes, arms, and feet. Occasionally, he would ask a question, such as, "Do you have pain here?" He put his hand precisely on the spot where Norman did indeed suffer a mysterious pain, for which no one yet could explain. Norman had not mentioned the pain and he was surprised to have Michio bring it up.

While Michio conducted his examination, Norman took the opportunity to examine Michio. He had a large head, straight black hair, a high forehead, and round, soft eyes. He had a wide nose and a tightly closed mouth. There was nothing about him that was affected or contrived, Norman later recalled. He was as natural and unselfconscious as any person Norman had ever met.

"I have prided myself on my judgment of character," Norman recalled years later. "The Ben Arnold Company employs more than 200 people and over the years I have dealt with a small army of employees. In addition, my experience in business has brought me into contact with all types, including strong men such as the one who now examined me. I sensed a gravity about Michio Kushi. Without making the slightest contrivance, he nevertheless radiated an air of substance and knowledge."

"You are nice people," Kushi began," but your diet and way of life has caused your disease," he said. "You have eaten too much fat, from steaks and other red meat, cheeses, and eggs. This, along with smoking and drinking, staying up too late, and working too hard, has caused your cancer."

"I've been told by my doctors that my cancer is incurable," Norman said.

Michio smiled. "What is medically impossible is macrobiotically possible. Your constitution is very strong. You can recover," he said.

Norman was inspired, to say the least. It wasn't just by Michio's words, he would later realize, but also by the fact that Michio was someone he trusted and respected. That's what gave credence and power to those words. Michio proceeded to outline the diet Norman should follow. It was composed chiefly of whole grains, such as brown rice, millet, barley, whole oats, corn, and buckwheat; fresh vegetables, especially leafy greens such as collard, kale, and mustard greens, and yellow vegetables such as squash and carrots; sea vegetables with names like hijiki, arame, nori, wakame, and kombu; beans, including azuki, navy, pinto, black, soy, and lentils; small amounts of the white meat of fish; and small amounts of fruit.

Michio encouraged Norman to walk regularly, and avoid all oils, fatty foods, refined flour products, sugar, and refined salt. Norman was to use high-quality sea salt and fermented soybean products, such as shoyu and tamari. He was to drink a small bowl of miso soup daily. (Miso, like tamari and shoyu, is a fermented soybean product that is made with rice, barley, or wheat.) Michio then encouraged him to wear only natural fabrics, and to take short brisk walks daily. He suggested that Norman pray before every meal and use a towel to scrub his body while he was in the shower. Michio said this would improve circulation and help the skin eliminate toxins. He told Norman to swim in the ocean, not a pool. Chlorine would sap minerals and strength that his body needed to overcome his illness, he said. He told him to listen to peaceful, inspiring music every day, and to fill his house with plants, which would pump oxygen into the air.

He then gave Norman one last bit of advice, which he thought was both funny and wise. "Every day, sing a happy song," he said. Norman and Gerry Sue laughed, but they knew what he meant. As Norman would say later, Michio had given him more hope and inspiration in the space of sixty minutes than all the doctors he had seen in his lifetime. Norman was elated.

"Michio," Norman began, "I've been very successful in business and I can be a generous fellow. I would like to be helpful to you by making a substantial contribution to your work." Michio looked at him warmly and said,

"When you get well, you'll help me help others." For Norman, that was the clincher. From that day on, Norman, Gerry Sue, and their three sons ate a macrobiotic diet.

Norman Arnold was a pillar within the Columbia community, with many social contacts, his synagogue being among the most important. That September also saw the arrival of the Jewish New Year, also known as Rosh Hashanah. Norman and Gerry Sue went to their synagogue where Norman read from the Torah, which he did every new year. Word of Norman's condition had spread quickly through Columbia, and that Rosh Hashanah service was filled with the weight of his approaching death. After Norman finished his reading, people from the congregation came up and embraced him, many with tears in their eyes. They were saying goodbye. Norman was moved. He, too, felt the tears begin to flow. Norman didn't know how to tell them that he wasn't out yet, and that he was going to fight this disease. As he returned to his pew, Gerry Sue leaned over to him and said, "What are they going to do next year when you're back?" Norman smiled and hugged his wife.

In 1982, Gerry Sue and Norman had been married twenty years and had been through many emotionally rocky times together. Norman's illness brought a whole new set of problems to their marriage. But instead of driving them apart, the illness brought them closer together. "You realize how important someone is when you are about to lose them," Gerry Sue said years later. "The love you have rises to the surface and you hold on to one another for dear life. At that point, you make the most of whatever time you have left together. If the time is spent searching for a cure, than that's what you do, but you're really loving each other as you do that." Gerry Sue poured her love into everything she did for Norman, including her cooking. In some mysterious and alchemical way, macrobiotics became like traditional chicken soup, the healing balm for all that ails a loved one.

That same September, Norman was given an injection of monoclonal antibodies. There would be only one injection. He would simply have to wait to see what effect the antibodies had, if any. That same month, Norman began taking the experimental chemotherapy protocol under Dr. Schein's direction. He underwent five treatments of chemotherapy. The effects of the drugs were devastating: weight loss, chronic fatigue, muscle wasting, nausea, and total loss of body hair. His weight dropped from 160 to 112 pounds. At times, he became despondent. By the time fall arrived, he wondered what good the chemotherapy might be doing for him, and why he was even subjecting himself to such treatment.

By Thanksgiving, Norman realized that he could not go on taking the chemotherapy. Dr. Schein had made it clear to him that the chemotherapy was not a cure; it wasn't even a guarantee of a few more months. But he wanted Norman to continue the chemotherapy on the chance that it might extend his life. Now Norman asked himself, what kind of life did chemotherapy offer? He was wasting away.

"I'd rather die in some more dignified way than have my sons remember me like this," Norman said. That month, he stopped the chemotherapy treatments.

Norman sought out many social and spiritual therapies that might be helpful. He and Gerry Sue attended the Carl Simonton Clinic in Dallas, Texas, where the two learned positive imaging techniques to treat the disease. Norman practiced the mind-body imaging techniques diligently. He also remained active in his synagogue and derived support from his spiritual community.

And then there was the social aspect of macrobiotic community. After finding other people in the area who practiced macrobiotics, Norman and Gerry Sue attended classes on cooking and macrobiotic philosophy. They also participated in pot luck dinners where other people shared their own healing stories. They visited large and vibrant macrobiotic communities in Florida and other southern states, where they received support. Both Norman and Gerry Sue remained in close contact with many of the people they met on these trips.

It wasn't long before the entire regimen was showing some results, not all of which were entirely reassuring. Initially, he lost more weight, which frightened both him and Gerry Sue. Michio told him that the weight loss was expected, and that he would gradually return to his optimal weight. Then Norman got a cold, which was more of a nuisance than anything else. This, too, was one of the ways the body was cleansing itself of toxins, Michio told him. But then Norman's tongue turned black, which shocked him and Gerry Sue. In a panic, they called Michio, who gave them the same response: This was a discharge of poisons from his liver and pancreas, and that it was, in fact, a good sign. His body was ridding itself of the cancer, Michio said. Norman was baffled and incredulous, but what could he do but wait and hope that Michio was right? Sure enough, within a few weeks, his tongue returned to a pink, healthy hue. He also started to regain some weight, which pleased him immensely. His face lost its formerly ghostly pallor and became clear and vibrant. And then his energy and overall strength increased dramatically. None of these were signs of advancing disease. On the contrary, Norman and Gerry Sue believed that Norman was turning things around.

On June 24, 1983, just nine months after he was diagnosed, Norman had another CT scan. This one showed only the faint presence of tumors in his pancreas and liver. Clearly, the cancer was in retreat. For the next six months, all of Norman's outward physical signs continued to improve. His doctors were amazed. None could explain what was happening to him, because none of them had seen such a restoration before. And then on December 22, 1983, Norman underwent yet another CT scan. This one was unequivocal: all clear. The test showed no signs of cancer anywhere in his body. Numerous other tests, including liver, blood, and ultrasound, confirmed the CT scan: Norman Arnold was free of cancer.

Thanks to the fact that he was followed closely by his medical doctors, Norman's healing journey was meticulously documented at every step. His case history, along with Marlene McKenna's and other remarkable and well-documented recovery stories, was presented to the National Cancer Institute's Committee for Alternative and Complementary Medicine. These case histories convinced the NCI committee that dietary changes warrant further study as adjunct treatments for cancer.

In 2000, Norman had been cancer-free for 18 years. Determined to have diet scientifically studied for its potential efficacy against cancer, Norman and Gerry Sue gave $10 million to the University of South Carolina School of Public Health, which was gifted to advance the study, teaching, and public education of nutrition. The School of Public Health was later renamed the Arnold School of Public Health. The Arnolds later gave another $7 million to the university to establish the Gerry Sue and Norman J. Arnold Institute on Aging, which was created to address childhood obesity, nutrition, stroke, and dementia, among other public health issues. In addition, Norman and Gerry Sue generously supported many charities and private individuals in need of help.

"Norman and Gerry Sue have always had high interest in improving the health status of vulnerable and disadvantaged populations, and they have backed that interest with major and frequent monetary gifts dispersed throughout the Columbia community and beyond," said Thomas Chandler, dean of the Arnold School of Public Health.

On August 16, 2016, Norman passed away peacefully at his home in Columbia, South Carolina, after being free of cancer for more than thirty-four years.

$\mathscr{E}$XPLORING
THE POSSIBILITIES

Every medical system throughout human history has been incomplete. By incomplete, I mean that essential aspects of the healing process have been ignored, misunderstood, or simply unknown to the system. In modern Western medicine, the missing part is *you*—or, to be more specific, your body's own healing forces. Yes, occasional references are made to boosting your immune system or preventing disease through proper diet and exercise, but when it comes to treating illness in earnest, medicine's arsenal is designed to act independently from whatever healing powers your body might possess. Hence, many common pharmaceuticals are used to force the body to behave differently–for example, drugs used to treat constipation, pain, or depression, or those used to lower blood pressure or cholesterol levels. Other medications are designed to kill the sources of certain illnesses—for example, antibiotics, which destroy bacteria, or chemotherapy agents, which are designed to kill cancer cells and tumors. In all of these cases, your body's healing forces are more or less irrelevant to the purpose and function of the pharmaceuticals used to treat disease.

Forcing the body to behave differently can result in a wide array of side effects, many of which can be severe or even life-threatening. In regard to the elimination of an illness, this approach can also lead to undesirable consequences. For one, the illness very often figures out ways to stay alive. Yes, antibiotics kill bacteria, but many strains mutate and become immune or resistant to antibiotic drugs, which is why illnesses that arise from antibiotic-resistant bacteria are far more difficult to treat. This phenomenon can also occur in cancer treatment. Chemotherapy does, indeed, kill many cancer cells, but, unfortunately, chemotherapy agents often fail to eradicate the cancer entirely. For many people, the remnants of the disease rekindle, and in time the disease rises from its ashes, oftentimes with a greater virulence than it had originally possessed. A recurrent cancer may be stronger, in part, because the surviving cancer cells have mutated in order to protect themselves against chemotherapy.

Complementary systems are also incomplete. Among their more obvious limitations is that these treatments often take time to show significant results. There is nothing in the complementary arsenal that can match medicine's emergency treatments, surgery, or psycho-pharmaceuticals for their immediate impacts on injury and illness. These and other medical treatments often save lives.

When it comes to life-threatening diseases, orthodox or modern medical treatments can often buy a patient time, but what you do with that time is up to you. For many, the added time is used to adopt a wide array of complementary treatments, which can make the difference between life and death. In order for complementary care to help restore health, however, two central goals must be achieved. The first is to reduce the body's overall toxic load, and thus starve the illness of what it needs to survive. The second is to follow a plant-based diet and other healing behaviors, which can dramatically boost your body's immune and healing forces. As you have read throughout this book, oftentimes these healing modalities are exactly what the body needs to overcome illness and restore health.

When we look a little closer at major diseases, it becomes clear why these two strategies can be effective. Heart disease is a good example of the effectiveness of the first strategy. By drastically lowering saturated fat and processed foods in the diet, blood cholesterol levels fall. This reduction of cholesterol can deprive the disorder of what it needs to sustain the plaques that clog the arteries to the heart. In time, these low cholesterol levels cause arterial plaques to shrink, restoring blood and oxygen flow to the heart and eliminating the disease.

Similar effects may be achieved with cancer. As described earlier in this book, specific changes in diet can dramatically lower insulin, inflammation, weight, elevated hormones, and many other problematic substances in the body, thus depriving some cancers of what they need to survive. The same is true of type-2 diabetes, metabolic syndrome, obesity, high blood pressure, and many other serious disorders.

This brings us to the second goal of complementary treatment: strengthening the body's healing forces, which include the immune system, antioxidant activity, and even gene function. Over the past five decades, research scientists have shown how complementary care can strengthen healing forces within the body. They have documented the importance of reducing stress and eating a plant-based diet. They have reported the healing effects of exercise, therapeutic touch, and community support. They have revealed the healing power of love, prayer, meditation, and faith. This information is essential, to be sure. And it is heartening to know that many hospitals and individual medical doctors have begun to incorporate more complementary forms of healing in their medical practices. But at this point, you should not expect a medical doctor to offer you a treatment protocol that includes natural ways to boost your healing forces, reduce your weight, lower your insulin levels, fight inflammation, or alter your gene function to improve your chances of recovery. You will have to take the initiative to look at the available information yourself and do your best to incorporate complementary practices along with your traditional medical care.

TRUE HEALING IS MORE THAN A PHYSICAL EVENT

Much of the conflict between medical and complementary care stems from their very different definitions of how health and illness are established and, on an even deeper level, what it means to be a human being. Medicine sees each person as essentially a biochemical machine—a complex machine, to be sure, but one that, above all else, is a material object. In this context, lab tests and computer-driven diagnostics have become the foundation of medical practice, simply because everything that is important in medicine is measurable. And because the body's own healing capacities are largely excluded from the modern medical approach, pharmaceutical drugs are used to alter biological processes and "manage" a disorder—and to keep on managing it through time, which is why, once you begin taking a prescription medication, chances are good that you are going to be on that drug for life. As time goes on and drug-related side effects arise, new prescriptions may be added to your regimen in order to manage these side effects of the original drug. In this scenario, there are no real cures and no true healing. There is only the management of symptoms. Medicine sees you through the lens of the intellectual center and leaves out what the intellectual mind regards as the chaotic and uncontrollable aspects of being human. It does not consider the healing power of love or the power of healing touch. It discounts the fact that the beneficial substances in plant foods work synergistically and cannot be reduced to a pill that will have the same effect as a plant-based diet.

Most complementary care systems define a human as a being composed of body, mind, heart, and spirit. Within the context of complementary care, all of aspects of humanity affect physical health, although not all of them are measurable with high-tech machines. In one way or another, complementary systems attempt to utilize the larger aspects of humanity to treat illness, which means that you are a crucial part of the healing process. In order to heal truly, you will have to embrace the more heart-centered aspects of your life—the parts of your nature that your doctor may reject as irrelevant to your illness. Yet it is through the synergy of the many mysterious powers within you that you may find a path to healing.

As you incorporate the seven steps outlined in this book into your daily life, you will begin to affect the most fundamental aspects of your humanity: your biology, diet, emotions, relationships, and even your spiritual life. As you address these aspects of your life, the way you think and feel about yourself and others, about life, and about the meaning of life's challenges will change. In short, you will transform your consciousness. According to most complementary healing systems, the "I" that you identify as yourself is more than your body, just as life is more than the physical objects you see with your eyes or detect with your other senses. And this "more" that you are—and the "more" that life is—is both true and essential, not only to the quality of your life, but also to the quantity.

THE SOUL AT THE HEART OF THE MATTER

Traditional healers, religious figures, and shamans throughout human history have asserted that all healing is ultimately a spiritual act—that the great learning is to align one's own awareness with the infinite intelligence that permeates and governs the universe. As this alignment is sustained, the individual realizes that, yes, physical changes are occurring, but also that something even deeper is being transformed. He or she begins to see the unity that all humans share with one another and with the source of life itself. For traditional healers and spiritual teachers alike, this evolution of consciousness has always been the most important aspect of healing, for the simple reason that sages of every tradition have maintained the idea that consciousness survives the body and continues on an infinite journey.

In the last century, scientists have attempted to bring a more rigorous approach to understanding the nature of consciousness and its relationship to the human body. The science of quantum physics has explored the connections between consciousness and the material world in great depth. Among its findings is that consciousness is not confined exclusively to the body but exists in a unified field of energy in which we are all joined. In this unified state, thoughts, feelings, and intentions, as forms of energy, pass through the medium of this field to affect the health and well-being of others, who, in the physical world, live at great distances but in the unified state are always connected to us. Not only does this view of a unified consciousness shatter our notions of space and time, but it also promises to transform deeply rooted fears about the temporary nature of life.

In the December 2001 issue of *The Lancet*, Dutch cardiologist Pim van Lommel reported on a study in which he and his colleagues interviewed 348 people who had survived cardiac arrest, but who had been considered clinically dead for extended periods of time. In other words, they could neither breathe nor circulate blood throughout their bodies and had no brain activity before eventually regaining consciousness and physical function. Van Lommel found that nearly one in five of these patients had had what has come to be known as a near-death experience. The characteristics of such an experience are now widely known. Upon coming back from presumed death, people report that they seemed to leave their bodies and were able to examine the events occurring around them from an elevated vantage point. They also mention having travelled through a tunnel that led to a bright light. Finally, they report having encountered relatives, friends, and a transcendent being who bathes them in unconditional love within this bright light.

One of the people interviewed in Van Lommel's study was a man who had suffered cardiac arrest and was pronounced clinically dead upon arriving at the hospital. While doctors were attempting to resuscitate him, a nurse removed the man's dentures so that a breathing tube could be inserted into his mouth. The doctors saved the man's life. Afterward, the man was placed in intensive care. Upon waking, he recognized the nurse who had removed his dentures and asked her to return his teeth. This request shocked the nurse because the man had been pronounced dead upon arrival at the hospital and had not regained consciousness while in the operating room. Indeed, he had lost brain function before the nurse had actually taken out his dentures. Van Lommel later asked the man how he had recognized the woman. He replied that when he had arrived in the operating room, he had experienced himself leaving his body and witnessing the events from a point above the operating table. Van Lommel realized that since the man had no brain function, he could neither have perceived these events nor hallucinated a fantasy that later proved remarkably accurate. Something other than the man's brain had observed these events.

Van Lommel speculated that consciousness might not necessarily be rooted in the brain but instead grounded in the body. Fifty billion of your cells die each day, yet your body continues to function as a whole, integrated, and coordinated unit. You do not perceive yourself as different even after all the cells of your body have been replaced. Van Lommel suggested that there might be some form of communication that coordinates cellular function and maintains the body's overall sense of itself. This communication might very well be what we think of as consciousness. If this is the case, consciousness would not arise from the brain, since many people lose all brain function while they are clinically dead.

Once again, we encounter the presence of an intelligence that directs communication within the body even as the body undergoes dramatic changes, such as experiencing the death of billions of cells each day. But clearly, Van Lommel's study and others like it suggest something more—that consciousness transcends the body and, indeed, doesn't need the body in order to go on living. Before his own death, macrobiotic educator Michio Kushi taught that, in the end, healing is a process by which we all come to understand the underlying nature of reality and the universe itself. "Consciousness lives on," Kushi asserted. "While we live here on earth, each of us is developing our new, unique constitution, which is our consciousness. That consciousness will be our new body that will be born into the world of spirit. We are developing that constitution on the basis of what we eat, how we think, and how we act toward each other." Kushi provided an illuminating insight for the stages of life. When you are in your mother's womb, he said, your body is nourished, supported, and developed within the watery confines of the amniotic sac. "The placenta allowed us to live in the world of water, while we developed a body that would live in the world of air," Kushi said. "Now that we live in the world of air, the physical body serves as an embryonic sac for our consciousness. The consciousness that we are growing now will be our new body when we are born into the world of vibration and energy."

INTIMATIONS OF IMMORTALITY

The healing modalities described in this book can help many people who are struggling with major illnesses prolong their lives and restore their states of health. These approaches can certainly improve the quality of your life by restoring love and joy to your daily existence. As you continue to walk this healing journey, you will begin to experience what Wordsworth called intimations of immortality—the subtle clues that your consciousness, your very soul, will one day be reunited with the source of life and love, and that the most true and fundamental aspects of life will never be destroyed.

$\mathcal{O}$NE DAY AT A TIME

After reading about all the healing methods presented in this book, you may be wondering how you might fit some of these ideas into an average day or even an average week. *How do I organize them into a regular routine?* you may be asking yourself. Actually, it's not as difficult as you might think. The first thing to do is to identity the new behaviors you want to adopt. Then you must practice them as consistently as possible—in some cases, every day; in others, once or twice a week. In this chapter, I present some of the most important healing methods described in this book and suggest at which times these practices may be incorporated into your daily schedule.

Among the practices you will want to adopt on a daily basis will be consumption of healing meals at breakfast, lunch, and dinner, along with health-promoting snacks and desserts. (See Recipes on page 181.) If you are pressed for time during the day, you may want to cook larger portions of whole grains, soups, or beans at night and then reheat them for lunches and dinners throughout the week. You can prepare fresh vegetables in fewer than ten minutes. Simply wash the veggies, chop them, add them to boiling water, and cook them for five to seven minutes, depending on the quantity desired. Alternatively, you can sauté them in water, or in olive or sesame oil.

Other healing activities that may be done on a daily basis include some type of spiritual practice or guided imagery, as well as some light exercise. Remember that physical exercise does not have to be done in a single thirty-minute session. Numerous studies have shown that three ten-minute exercise sessions can provide greater health benefits than a single thirty-minute workout, so don't refrain from that walk just because it will take "only" ten minutes to complete. Do three ten-minute walks each day—one in the morning, another at lunch, and one more in the afternoon or evening—and feel the health benefits add up.

In addition to these daily behaviors, you may want to do certain activities periodically throughout the week. These may include doing volunteer work; seeing a healer, therapist, counselor, or acupuncturist; or participating in a support group. I have made suggestions for when you could engage in these periodic activities, but these recommended times can be moved around to suit your own specific schedule.

MORNING

After you get out of bed in the morning and before you eat breakfast, try your best to engage in a short spiritual practice. Choose one or another of the spiritual practices described in step six (see page 101), or do some other practice that inspires you. Consider combining spiritual practices, such as a short period of meditation followed by reading sacred literature and engaging in prayer.

If you are new to these practices, you may want to limit the amount of time you dedicate to them. The more arduous you make such activities— especially at the beginning of the healing process—the less likely you are to stay with them. In other words, don't worry about the length of time you spend meditating but rather focus on meditating consistently. Consistency is power. If you use a particular practice for only five minutes a day, you will benefit. Through consistency, you will naturally extend the amount of time you sit in meditation or in prayer or reading, without having to use much discipline. Among the most important factors to consider, especially at the outset, is to give yourself time to get comfortable with the various practices, to feel which ones work best for you, and then commit to these practice so that you can experience their positive effects on your body, mind, heart, and spirit. The more you do them, the more you will enjoy them. In time, you will come to rely on your practices to create stability and balance in your life.

If you are new to meditation, or have been using other spiritual practices and want to start meditating, consider doing just five minutes of watching your breath every morning. (See page 19 for instructions.) The same holds for prayer, especially if sitting in meditation or prayer every morning is new to you. Longer meditation or prayer sessions are not necessarily better. Sincerity, concentration, silencing your mind, and a sense of connection with a higher power are what matter.

Some days, you may not feel anything from your practices. Other days you may feel so connected to your heart, inner life, and the source of your life that you may be moved to tears. Try not to evaluate any practice on the basis of your emotional state. Rather, stay committed to your meditation or prayer routine. Empty your mind in meditation. Concentrate on the words and feelings in prayer. Let each practice bring you peace and balance. Meanwhile, let the intelligence that flows within you do its work, with or without your conscious recognition.

Prayer can be the recitation of a formal prayer from your religious tradition, or simply the act of talking to the Creator about what you are feeling and the events that are taking place in your life. If you choose to chant, chant for five to fifteen minutes at each session. You can also listen to recordings or watch videos of other people chanting and chant along with them. Such a practice can be very powerful and uplifting. If you choose to find healing in spiritual writings, you can read any spiritually inspiring book or sacred text you wish, such as the Bible, the Vedas, the Bhagavad Gita, or the Koran.

If you decide to write in a journal each morning, try to limit yourself to three pages, unless of course you are so full of memories, thoughts, ideas, and feelings that you must get them all on the page. If that's the case, let it all pour out. But just as with other spiritual practices, more is not necessarily better. Write what is true; that's more important than the number of pages written.

When you write, try to express those feelings that exist below the surface of your awareness. Don't worry about grammar or spelling. Don't censor yourself. Just write your feelings in whatever terms that come to mind. Release your rage, fear, sadness. Explain the details of your pain. What is most important is that you arrive at compassion for all you have been through in life. Compassion, you will recall, is not self-pity. The former is a form of love; the latter is infused with self-criticism and self-loathing, both of which are very destructive to your health.

If you will be combining similar practices, such as meditation and prayer, five minutes of each will be sufficient. If you will be using different types of practices together—for example, meditation, prayer, and journal writing—allow fifteen to forty minutes in total per session.

BREAKFAST

The following is a general meal plan recommendation for breakfast. See the recipes at the end of this book for more specific suggestions. (See Recipes on page 217.)

Start with a simple miso soup. After preparing the broth from your miso paste, the soup can include any of the following vegetables: wakame seaweed; roots such as carrots, parsnip, or daikon; or green vegetables such as broccoli, kale, bok choy, or Chinese cabbage. Along with the soup, try a cooked grain. Make sure the grain is well cooked and soft. Ideal breakfast grains include steel cut oats, brown rice, and quinoa. In addition, a green or leafy vegetable such as broccoli, collard greens, kale, bok choy, or watercress would go well with your grain. As for tea, drink bancha, kukicha, chamomile, or some other non-caffeinated herbal tea made with spring water. If your health permits, you can also drink a grain coffee substitute, such as Dandy or Pero.

After breakfast, you may engage in ten to thirty minutes of light exercise, such as light stretching, walking, yoga, stationary bicycling, dancing (slow, conscious, rhythmic movement), or practicing a martial art.

LATE MORNING

Between 10:30 AM and 11 AM, have a light snack, such as a cup of vegetable soup. If you are at work at this time, bring it in an insulated container. Alternatively, you could have a piece of fruit, such as an apple or pear, or a cup of berries. Fruit may be cooked or fresh. A handful of roasted sunflower or pumpkin seeds and raisins is a good option as well.

You might also consider reading a short passage from sacred or uplifting literature. Suggestions include excerpts from the Bible, such as passages from Psalms, the Book of Proverbs, the Gospels, or the Epistles of Paul; poems by Hafiz, Rumi, or St. Francis; or any other source of spiritual writing. You could also write one to three pages in a journal, allowing yourself to release your uncensored feelings and thoughts. If you did not exercise earlier, you could perform some light exercise at this point, such as a short walk.

Finally, you could write an encouraging letter to someone in need of support, call a friend and focus on your friend's concerns, or pray for someone who is ill or struggling in some way.

On Any Given Day

If possible, once a week, see a counselor or therapist, a massage practitioner, an acupuncturist, or some other form of complementary healer. In addition, do volunteer work. If you are able, reach out and find a way to support others.

LUNCH

Suggestions for lunch include a cooked grain such as brown rice, quinoa, or millet, or a high-quality pasta such as udon, buckwheat (soba), or spaghetti. Add to this base a green vegetable or root vegetable (boiled, steamed, or sautéed), or some leafy greens. As a beverage, have water or herbal tea, and finish off your meal with a piece of fruit, preferably cooked.

After lunch, take a ten-minute walk. If possible, sit quietly and concentrate on your breath for five minutes. You could also write in your journal if there are thoughts you'd like to express. If you are dealing with anxiety, or if you have experienced some difficult situation or conflict during the day, writing can be especially grounding.

LATE AFTERNOON

By late afternoon, feel free to enjoy a light snack of lightly roasted seeds or nuts and raisins. Follow it with a short reading of inspiring literature, sacred literature, or poetry, and then do some gentle exercise for a few minutes. As these suggestions are optional, you may engage in one or all of these activities, following the path that feels right to you.

DINNER

Similar to the other meals of the day, good options for dinner include vegetable soup, a cooked grain, cooked beans (e.g., black beans, chickpeas, mung beans, aduki beans), cooked green and leafy vegetables, and cooked root or sweet vegetables. If you are looking for variety, cooked whitefish is also a menu possibility.

EVENING

Once evening has arrived, get out your journal again. Write at least ten things that happened over the course of the day for which you are grateful. Was there an improvement in some aspect of your health? Did someone support you or engage you with kindness? Did you enjoy your food? Is there something about your environment that you really love? Did someone make you smile or laugh? Did you experience and express feelings of love for those most important to you? Alternatively, you could write at least ten things that you love about yourself and life.

Your goal for the rest of the night is to enjoy yourself. Watch a funny movie, read an absorbing novel, listen to some great music, be with loved ones. Do your best to enjoy some part of your evening. If weather permits, go for a walk. Marvel at your surroundings. If you are able to walk in nature, look at the trees, the grass, the sky; smell the air; find the beauty that surrounds you and receive it in your heart and soul. Beauty offers a unique healing gift. If you live in the city, appreciate the architecture of the buildings; watch the people on the street without the slightest judgment; greet people with warmth and caring; appreciate all the work and talent that went into creating such a place in which so many people can live and work. Open up to and appreciate the beauty in all that surrounds you. If you'd like, do a short meditation or prayer session (five to ten minutes) before going to bed.

TRANSFORMATIONAL TOOLS

With just a little time, focus, and dedication, the practices you choose to incorporate into your daily schedule will start to have a profound effect on your health, outlook, and overall life. They are powerful, transformational tools. Use them daily and experience the opening of your heart, the relaxation of your mind, and the healing of your body.

RECIPES

$\mathcal{D}$IETARY RECOMMENDATIONS

The recommendations and recipes provided in this chapter are intended for people who have been diagnosed with a serious illness and want to use a healing diet as part of their recovery programs. A week's worth of menu plans are provided to offer healthful ideas for breakfasts, lunches, and dinners. Also included are options for snacks and desserts. First, let's begin with some general guidelines in regard to quality food choices.

Gluten is a protein in some grains and grain products that can be harmful to many people. It seems as though gluten is a food substance best avoided if you are attempting to heal from a serious illness. This book has taken into account the growing awareness of gluten sensitivity and has excluded this protein from all recommended foods and recipes. In addition, this book urges you to eat only organically grown grains, vegetables, beans, and fruit, and to eat only ocean-caught white fish. Organic plant foods have been grown without the use of synthetic fertilizers, pesticides, or herbicides. Synthetic fertilizers and pesticides may be harmful and should be avoided in a healing diet. Organic meat comes from animals that have been raised only on organic plant foods and are free of synthetic hormones, antibiotics, or artificial coloring agents. As well, be sure that the food you eat is non-GMO (genetically modified organism), as GMO crops have been genetically designed to tolerate synthetic pesticides and may be sprayed with unusually high amounts of these chemicals.

As far as salt is concerned, only high-quality sea salt—such as Celtic gray sea salt or Himalayan pink salt—is recommended. Both are rich in a wide array of trace minerals that are essential to health and healing. Standard table salt is highly refined, lacking in trace minerals, and will even contain sugar to stabilize the added iodide. For those who have allergies to soybeans and soy products, the soups, stews, and sauces found in this book may be made with sea-salt or Himalayan salt instead of miso, tamari, or shoyu. In terms of oil, only organic cold-pressed extra virgin olive oil, organic sesame oil, and organic toasted sesame oil are recommended for use in cooking. While on a healing diet, limit oil to 1 tablespoon daily.

Avoid all processed food and sugar while you are combating major illness. Virtually all processed foods contain sugar today, though the food industry has become more adept at hiding the sugar under various chemical names. Cut out artificial sweeteners, such as aspartame and NutraSweet, as well. There are also a variety of "natural" sweeteners that should be avoided, including agave, date sugar, honey, and maple syrup. Until you have restored and stabilized your health—meaning you have been healthy for more than a year—cease consumption of all types of sugar, whether synthetic or natural.

Try not to overeat. Quantity can affect the quality of the food and its effects on your body, Michio Kushi used to say. As a general rule, eat until you are about 80-percent full. Leave a little room so that your stomach and intestines can easily digest your food. Chew every mouthful at least thirty-five times, preferably fifty times. Follow the wonderful advice of Mahatma Gandhi, who used to say, "Drink your food and chew your soup." Sit down and enjoy every meal. Give your food your full attention. Try to avoid standing while eating. Consider offering a prayer of thanks before you eat. It should center your body and mind, and prepare you to receive your food in a state of gratitude. Finally, stop eating three hours before bed. Avoid going to bed on a full stomach.

WHOLE GRAINS

Eat a cooked whole grain at every meal. The portion of grain you eat per meal should make up approximately one-third to one-fourth of your plate at each sitting. In addition, include a high-quality gluten-free pasta in your meal plan once a week.

Recommended grains include brown rice, wild rice, quinoa, millet, steel-cut oats, buckwheat, amaranth, and teff. Boiling is the preferred method for cooking a grain, although it may also be pressure cooked, steamed, or sautéed. Gluten-free pasta may be made from whole grains, including brown rice, quinoa, and corn. (If you use corn pasta, make sure the corn is non-GMO.)

VEGETABLES AND LEGUMES

Eat at least three servings of green or leafy vegetables every day, such as bok choy, broccoli, collard greens, kale, leeks, mustard greens, Chinese cabbage, green cabbage, or watercress. Make sure to eat a green or leafy vegetable at every meal, including breakfast. Eat two or three servings of round or sweet vegetables daily. Included in this group are onions, parsnips, rutabaga, squash, turnips, and sweet potatoes. (Avoid white potatoes, as they raise insulin levels.) Eat two servings per day of root vegetables, such as burdock, carrots, daikon radish, lotus root, parsnips, red radish, rutabaga, or turnips. Eat shiitake, reishi, maitake, *Coriolis versicolor* (also known as turkey tail), or button mushrooms four times each week. Eat a white vegetable four to six times per week. These include daikon, onion, cauliflower, and turnip.

Make vegetables approximately 60 percent of your daily food intake. The vast majority of your vegetables–90 percent—should be cooked. Avoid highly acidic vegetables, such as tomatoes and eggplant, which drain minerals from the blood and require additional work from the kidneys in order to alkalize the blood. Eat a small serving (2 tablespoons) of sea vegetables per day. If possible, eat a bowl of vegetable-rich soup in miso broth five to seven times a week. Include some form of seaweed, green, or root vegetable in the soup. Lastly, eat one serving of whole beans daily. Preferred beans include aduki beans, black beans, garbanzo beans, lentils, mung beans, navy beans, pinto beans, and white beans.

FISH

Make white fish your singular source of animal protein. White fish is low in fat and therefore low in all the problematic substances commonly found in other types of fish. Eat white fish two or more times per week. The serving size should be approximately 3 ounces, or about the size of a deck of cards.

OTHER TIPS

In addition to miso soup, eat some form of probiotic food daily. Recommended probiotic-rich items include sauerkraut (1 to 2 tablespoons), kimchee, natto, tempeh, and a variety of pickled vegetables. Drink spring water throughout the day. If spring water cannot be found, drink filtered water. In addition to water, drink non-aromatic teas. Healthful teas include chamomile, rooibos, bancha, kukicha, and peppermint. If caffeine can be tolerated, green and black teas are recommended. Avoid all coffee. If you would like a coffee-like beverage, drink a high-quality grain coffee substitute such as Pero, Cafix, Inka, or Dandy.

Eat fruit sparingly because of its high sugar content. Preferred fruit includes apples, pears, berries, and, when in season, watermelon. Try to eat fruit that grows in your own climate. If you live in a temperate climate, avoid tropical fruit. Whenever possible, cook your fruit to make compote. Eat a small amount of nuts and seeds—about the amount that would fit in the palm of your hand—three to five times a week. Soak nuts and seeds overnight to increase their digestibility. Preferred nuts are almonds, Brazil nuts, chestnuts (used mostly in cooking whole grains such as brown rice), pistachios, and walnuts. Preferred seeds include chia, flax (grind before using), pumpkin, sesame (both yellow and black), and sunflower. When looking for a snack or dessert, remember these numerous options.

SOUPS

RED LENTIL SOUP

SERVINGS: 4 to 6

• •

7 cups water	3 tablespoons dark gluten-free miso, or to taste, diluted in small amount of soup stock
I cup red lentils, washed and drained	
I large onion, diced	I cup chopped scallions or fresh parsley
2 medium carrots, diced	
2 beets, diced	

1. In a $4^{1}/_{2}$-quart saucepan, combine the water, lentils, onion, carrots, and beets. Bring to a boil and then lower the heat to simmer. Cover and cook for at least 1 hour. Remove from heat. Blend ingredients until smooth.

2. Add the miso to the saucepan, return to low heat, and cook for 5 to 10 minutes. Do not boil the miso. Garnish with the scallions or parsley and serve.

DRIED MUSHROOM AND SPINACH SOUP

SERVINGS: 4 to 6

7 cups water	1 onion, diced
2 cups dried mushrooms, any type	1 carrot, diced
4 cups spinach	Tamari to taste

1. In a $4^1/_2$-quart saucepan, boil the water and add the dried mushrooms. Lower the heat to simmer and cook for approximately 20 minutes, or until tender.

2. Add the spinach, onion, and carrot to the saucepan. Cover and simmer for 15 minutes. Add more water if needed. Add the tamari, simmer for 10 minutes, and serve.

MINESTRONE SOUP

SERVINGS: 4 to 6

12 cups water, divided	2 small winter squash, cubed
1 cup dried kidney beans, soaked overnight and drained	2 potatoes, diced
1 strip kelp	1 teaspoon rosemary
3 onions, chopped	1 teaspoon basil
3 carrots, chopped	2 cups gluten-free macaroni
3 stalks celery, sliced	3 tablespoons dark gluten-free miso, or to taste, diluted in $^1/_2$ cup soup stock
3 cloves garlic, sliced	1 cup chopped fresh parsley

1. In a $4^1/_2$-quart saucepan, combine 6 cups of the water, kidney beans, and kelp. Bring to a boil and then lower the heat to simmer. Cook for $1^1/_2$ hours, or until beans are tender. Drain the beans.

2. In a 6-quart stockpot, combine the onion, carrots, celery, garlic, squash, potatoes, rosemary, basil, and 6 cups of the water. Bring to a boil and then lower the heat to medium. Cook for 20 minutes, or until vegetables are soft. Add the macaroni and miso. Lower the heat to simmer for 10 minutes. Do not boil miso. Garnish with the parsley and serve.

SQUASH SOUP

SERVINGS: 4 to 6

• •

6 cups of water

8 cups cubed winter squash

I large sweet potato, cubed

2 tablespoons dark gluten-free miso, or to taste, diluted in $^1/_2$ cup soup stock

Freshly grated ginger to taste

1. In a $4^1/_2$-quart saucepan, combine the squash and sweet potato and water. Bring to boil and then lower the heat to simmer. Cook for 1 hour, or until vegetables are soft. Add more water if needed. Remove from heat. Blend ingredients until smooth.

2. Add the miso to the saucepan, return to low heat, and cook for 5 to 10 minutes. Do not boil miso. Add the ginger and serve.

SIMPLE MISO SOUP

SERVINGS: 2 to 4

• •

$^1/_2$ cup finely chopped alaria or wild Atlantic wakame, soaked overnight

5 cups water

I cup carrot matchsticks

2 tablespoons gluten-free miso, or to taste, diluted in $^1/_2$ cup soup stock

5 scallions, thinly sliced

$^1/_2$ teaspoon freshly grated ginger

1. In a $4^1/_2$-quart saucepan, combine the alaria and water (including soaking water). Bring to a boil. Cook on high heat for 30 minutes.

2. Lower the heat to simmer. Add the carrot to saucepan, cover, and simmer for 10 minutes. Add the miso to the soup and simmer for 10 minutes. Do not boil miso. Add the scallions, ginger, and serve.

Helpful Tip

There are many ways to make simple miso soup. Feel free to experiment by using other vegetables.

WATERCRESS SOUP

SERVINGS: 4 to 6

• •

7 cups water	6 tablespoons dark gluten-free miso, or to taste, diluted in $^1/_2$ cup soup stock
2 small onions, chopped	
4 bunches watercress	

1. In a $4^1/_2$-quart saucepan, combine the water, onions, and watercress. Bring to a boil. Lower the heat to medium and cook for 30 minutes, or until vegetables are soft. Add more water if needed. Remove from heat. Blend ingredients until smooth.

2. Add the miso, return to low heat, simmer for 10 minutes, and serve.

CURRIED CAULIFLOWER SOUP

SERVINGS: 4 to 6

• •

I head cauliflower	I teaspoon curry powder
Olive oil	$^1/_2$ teaspoon ground cumin
Pinch sea salt	$^1/_4$ teaspoon coriander
I onion, diced	$^1/_8$ teaspoon ground cinnamon
2 carrots, diced	8 cups water
I stalk celery, diced	2 tablespoons gluten free miso, or to taste, diluted in $^1/_2$ cup soup stock

1. Preheat oven to 400°F.

2. Place the cauliflower in glass dish or cast iron skillet and coat with the olive oil and sea salt. Bake for 30 minutes, or until soft.

3. In a $4^1/_2$-quart saucepan, combine the cauliflower, onion, carrots, celery, curry powder, cumin, coriander, and cinnamon. Add the water and bring to a boil. Lower the heat to simmer, cover, and cook for 1 hour. Remove from heat. Blend ingredients until smooth.

4. Add the miso, return to low heat, simmer for 10 minutes, and serve.

SHIITAKE MUSHROOM AND QUINOA SOUP

SERVINGS: 4 to 6

7 cups water

$1/2$ cup quinoa, rinsed

10 shiitake mushrooms, soaked for twenty minutes, thinly sliced

1 onion, diced

2 carrots, diced

7 leaves Chinese cabbage, sliced into small pieces

3 tablespoons gluten-free miso, or to taste, diluted in $1/2$ cup soup stock

1 scallion, sliced

1 teaspoon freshly grated ginger

1. In a $4^1/_2$-quart saucepan, combine the water, quinoa, and shiitake mushrooms. Bring to a boil and then lower the heat to simmer. Add the onion, carrots, and Chinese cabbage. Add more water if needed. Cover and cook for 1 hour.

2. Add the miso and simmer for 10 minutes. Garnish with the scallion and ginger and serve.

WHITEFISH SOUP

SERVINGS: 4 to 6

6 cups water

1 strip kelp

1 pound whitefish fillet, left whole

2 cups sliced leeks

1 cup chopped Chinese cabbage

1 cup diced carrots

1 teaspoon sea salt

Tamari to taste

$1/2$ teaspoon freshly grated ginger

1 cup chopped fresh parsley

1. In a $4^1/_2$-quart saucepan, combine the water and kelp. Bring to a boil. Lower the heat to medium and cook for 10 minutes.

2. Lower the heat to simmer and add the whitefish, leeks, cabbage, carrots, and sea salt. Add more water if needed. Cook for 30 minutes.

3. Remove the kelp, cut into small pieces, and return it to the soup. Season with the tamari and simmer for 5 minutes. Add the ginger, garnish with the parsley, and serve.

WHOLE GRAINS

OATMEAL

SERVINGS: 2 to 4

• •

5 cups water

I cup steel-cut oats, rinsed well

Pinch sea salt

Handful raisins

I tablespoon ground roasted flax seeds or chia seeds

1. In a 4$\frac{1}{2}$-quarter saucepan, combine the water, steel-cut oats, sea salt, and raisins. Bring to a boil. Lower the heat to simmer, cover, and cook for 30 minutes.

2. Garnish with the flax seeds and serve. Top with blueberries or cranberries if desired.

BUCKWHEAT AND MACARONI

SERVINGS: 4 to 6

• •

2 cups buckwheat groats

8 cups water

Pinch sea salt

I onion, minced

2 tablespoons olive oil

$\frac{1}{2}$ pound gluten-free macaroni, cooked

Tamari to taste

I teaspoon mustard (optional)

$\frac{1}{2}$ cup chopped fresh parsley

1. In a small skillet, toast the buckwheat for 5 minutes.

2. In a 4$\frac{1}{2}$-quart saucepan, combine the buckwheat, water, and sea salt. Bring to a boil and cook for 30 minutes, or until buckwheat is soft and the water has been absorbed. Remove from heat.

3. In a large skillet, sauté the onion in the olive oil for 5 to 7 minutes, or until soft. Add the buckwheat, macaroni, tamari, and mustard. Mix well. Garnish with the parsley and serve.

SIMPLE BROWN RICE

SERVINGS: 4 to 6

• •

2 cups brown rice, rinsed and
soaked overnight in 3 cups water
(discard soaking water)

6 cups water

Pinch sea salt

1. In a 4$^1/_2$-quart saucepan, combine the rice, water, and sea salt. Bring to a boil. Lower the heat to simmer, cover, and cook for 45 minutes.

2. Drain off any excess water and simmer, covered, for 5 minutes more.

MILLET AND CAULIFLOWER

SERVINGS: 2 to 4

• •

7 cups water

I cup millet

I onion, diced

$^1/_2$ cauliflower,
broken up into small pieces

Pinch sea salt

I clove garlic

1. In a 4$^1/_2$-quart saucepan, combine the water, millet, onion, cauliflower, sea salt, and garlic. Bring to a boil. Lower the heat to simmer, cover, and cook for 45 minutes, or until the vegetables are tender.

2. Mash with a potato masher for a creamy consistency. (Cooked millet really soaks up the water after it sits awhile.)

GREEK SPIRALS

SERVINGS: 4 to 6

• •

3 tablespoons olive oil

I onion, diced

10 button mushrooms, diced

10 cups spinach, cut small

5 black olives, chopped small

I teaspoon minced garlic

6 cups gluten-free noodles, cooked

Tamari to taste

1. In a large skillet, sauté the onion, mushrooms, spinach, olives, and garlic in the olive oil.

2. When the vegetables are soft, mix in the noodles. Add the tamari and serve.

JAPANESE FRIED RICE

SERVINGS: 4 to 6

2 tablespoons sesame oil

3 cloves garlic, minced

1 onion, diced

2 carrots, thinly sliced

1 stalk broccoli,
cut into small florets

2 stalks celery, thinly sliced

3 cups cooked brown rice

2 tablespoons tamari

1 teaspoon freshly grated ginger

3 scallions, thinly sliced

1 sheet sushi nori

1. In a large skillet, sauté the garlic in the sesame oil for 3 minutes. Add the onion, carrots, broccoli, and celery. Sauté for 5 minutes.

2. Add the rice and tamari. Mix well. Cook for 5 minutes. Turn off the heat and add the ginger and scallions. Mix well. Garnish with torn pieces of the sushi nori.

NOODLES WITH SAUCE

SERVINGS: 2 to 4

$1/_2$ pound gluten-free noodles of your choice, cooked

$1/_4$ cup tamari

2 tablespoons sesame oil

1 tablespoon toasted sesame oil

1 tablespoon apple cider vinegar

1 teaspoon freshly grated ginger

1 teaspoon chopped garlic

1 cup chopped scallions

1 tablespoon toasted sesame seeds

1. In a small mixing bowl, combine the tamari, vinegar, oils, ginger, and garlic.

2. Mix and pour over the noodles. Add the scallions and seeds. Toss and serve.

QUINOA SALAD

SERVINGS: 2 to 4

2 cups water

Pinch sea salt

1 cup quinoa, rinsed

$^1/_4$ Bermuda onion, diced

$^1/_2$ cucumber, peeled and diced

1 carrot, diced

Tamari to taste

Olive oil to taste

Lemon juice to taste

1. In a $4^1/_2$-quart saucepan, combine the water and sea salt. Bring to a boil. Lower the heat to simmer, add the quinoa, cover, and cook for approximately 30 minutes.

2. Add the onion, cucumber, carrot, tamari, olive oil, and lemon juice. Fluff with a fork, toss, and serve.

PESTO SAUCE FOR PASTA

SERVINGS: 2 to 4

2 cups basil leaves

2 cloves garlic, minced

2 tablespoons walnuts,
soaked overnight

$^1/_2$ cup olive oil

$^1/_4$ cup water

Tamari to taste

1. In a blender, combine the basil leaves, garlic, walnuts, olive oil, water, and tamari.

2. Blend until smooth, making adjustments to suit your taste. Pour over your favorite noodles.

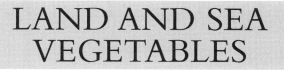

LAND AND SEA VEGETABLES

BAKED WINTER SQUASH

SERVINGS: 2 to 4

I acorn squash or any winter squash   Olive oil

1. Preheat oven to 375°F.

2. Wash off any dirt on the rind of the squash and then cut the squash in half. Remove the seeds.

3. On a large baking sheet, place squash halves sliced side down and bake for about 1 hour. Lightly coat with olive oil and serve.

BAKED ROOT STEW

SERVINGS: 4 to 6

Any combination of carrots, onions, rutabagas, daikon radishes, parsnips, leeks, or sweet potatoes

Olive oil

Balsamic vinegar

Tamari

1. Preheat oven to 350°F.

2. Chop the vegetables into very small pieces.

3. In a Dutch oven, spread the vegetables evenly, drizzle the olive oil and balsamic vinegar over the vegetables, finishing the dish off with a few drops of the tamari. Bake for 2 hours, or until vegetables are soft. Serve.

BAKED SWEET POTATOES

SERVINGS: 4 to 6

3 sweet potatoes, washed,
cut in half lengthwise

Olive oil

Garlic powder to taste

Sea salt to taste

Black pepper to taste

1. Preheat oven to 350°F.

2. Place the sweet potatoes cut sides down in a glass dish or cast iron skillet. Lightly coat with the olive oil, garlic, sea salt, and pepper. Bake for $1^{1}/_{2}$ hours, or until tender inside. (If you would like the potatoes to have crunchier skins, turn the oven up to 400°F for the last 30 minutes of baking.)

LUSCIOUS LEEKS

SERVINGS: 4 to 6

2 cups water

5 to 6 leeks, sliced
(1-inch slices)

1 carrot, diced

1 teaspoon tamari

3 teaspoons mustard

1 teaspoon balsamic vinegar

3 teaspoons olive oil

1. In a $4^{1}/_{2}$-quart saucepan, combine the water, leeks, carrot, and tamari. Bring to a boil. Lower the heat to simmer, cover, and cook for approximately 25 minutes, or until tender. Remove cover and continue cooking until no liquid remains.

2. Combine the mustard, balsamic vinegar, and olive oil in a covered jar. Shake the jar well. Pour mixture over the vegetables and serve.

RUTABAGA AND DILL

SERVINGS: 4 to 6

2 large rutabagas,
cut into chunks

2 tablespoons tamari

2 tablespoons dried dill

1. In a 4$^1/_2$-quart saucepan, cover the rutabaga chunks with water. Add the tamari and dill. Bring to a boil.

2. Lower the heat to simmer. Cook for approximately 1 hour, or until rutabaga chunks are soft and liquid is almost gone.

RATATOUILLE

SERVINGS: 4 to 6

2 tablespoons sesame oil

1 onion, sliced

2 cloves garlic, minced

3 large yellow summer squash, sliced

2 zucchini, sliced

1 teaspoon sea salt

$^1/_2$ cup water

1. In a large skillet, sauté the onion and garlic in the sesame oil for 3 minutes.

2. Add the yellow summer squash, zucchini, and sea salt. Add the water and stir. Cover and simmer until vegetables are tender.

CHINESE VEGETABLES

SERVINGS: 4 to 6

2 tablespoons sesame oil

1 clove garlic, grated

1 large onion, sliced

4 cups thinly sliced cabbage

1 large carrot, chopped

1 cup snow peas, ends removed

2 scallions, sliced

$^1/_2$ tablespoon apple cider vinegar

1 tablespoon tamari

1 teaspoon freshly grated ginger

1 cup almonds, soaked overnight and roasted

1. In a large skillet, sauté the garlic and onion in the sesame oil for 3 minutes. Add the cabbage, carrot, snow peas, and scallions. Raise the heat to high and cook until tender but still crunchy, stirring frequently.

2. Lower the heat to simmer, cover, and cook for 3 minutes. Add the tamari, ginger juice, and apple cider vinegar. Stir well. Sprinkle the roasted almonds over the vegetables and serve.

SAUTÉED LEAFY GREENS

SERVINGS: 2 to 4

1 tablespoon olive oil

2 cloves garlic, minced

3 drops tamari

1 bunch leafy greens (kale, collards, mustard greens, broccoli, or any other leafy green), chopped

1. In a large skillet, sauté the garlic in the olive oil for 3 minutes.

2. Add the leafy greens and tamari. Sauté for 5 to 7 minutes. Serve.

MIXED GREENS

SERVINGS: 2 to 4

1 tablespoon olive oil

2 scallions, sliced

4 cloves garlic, minced

1 cup chopped spinach

1 cup chopped watercress

1 cup chopped kale

1 cup chopped Swiss chard

1. In a large skillet, sauté the scallions and garlic in the olive oil for 5 minutes, or until soft.

2. Add the spinach, watercress, kale, and Swiss chard. Sauté for 15 minutes, or until tender. Serve.

BABY BOK CHOY WITH YAMS AND GINGER

SERVINGS: 4 to 6

2 tablespoons olive oil

1 small garnet yam, thinly sliced

2 scallions

1 teaspoon freshly grated ginger

5 heads baby bok choy, halved, bases removed

1 tablespoon tamari

Juice of 1 lemon

1. In a large skillet, sauté the yam in the olive oil for 5 minutes. Cover and cook for 2 minutes, or until tender.

2. Add the scallions and ginger. Sauté for 1 minute. Add the baby bok choy and tamari (add a little water if needed) and sauté until soft. Pour the lemon juice over the vegetables and serve.

INDIAN VEGETABLE CURRY

SERVINGS: 4 to 6

2 tablespoons sesame oil	I tablespoon dried curry blend
I onion, diced	2 teaspoons freshly grated ginger
2 cloves garlic, minced	2 cups chopped broccoli
I teaspoon cumin	2 cups chopped cauliflower
I teaspoon sea salt	$^1/_2$ cup chopped carrot
$^1/_2$ teaspoon black pepper	$^1/_2$ green peas, fresh or frozen

1. In a large skillet, sauté the onion and garlic in the sesame oil for 5 minutes, or until soft. Add the cumin, sea salt, pepper, curry blend, and ginger. Sauté for 1 minute.

2. Add the broccoli, cauliflower, carrot, and peas. Sauté for 15 minutes (add a little water if needed), or until tender. Serve.

BOILED LEAFY GREENS

SERVINGS: 2 to 4

I bunch leafy greens (kale, collards, mustard greens, broccoli, or other dark green), chopped	Pinch sea salt
	4 drops toasted sesame oil
	4 drops tamari

1. In a $4^1/_2$-quart saucepan, cover the greens with water and bring to a boil. Boil for 3 to 5 minutes.

2. Drain and rinse the greens. Serve with dressing of your choice.

SALADS, PICKLES, CONDIMENTS, SAUCES, AND DRESSINGS

CUCUMBER, ALARIA, AND WATERCRESS SALAD

SERVINGS: 4 to 6

I cup finely chopped alaria or wild Atlantic wakame, soaked overnight

5 cups water

6 tablespoons apple cider vinegar

I tablespoon toasted sesame oil

$1^1/_2$ tablespoons water

3 tablespoons tamari

3 cucumbers, julienned

3 bunches watercress, cut into small pieces

1. In a $4^1/_2$-quart saucepan, combine the alaria and water (including soaking water). Bring to a boil. Cook on high heat for 30 minutes. Remove from heat and drain.

2. In a mixing bowl, combine the apple cider vinegar, sesame oil, water, and tamari. Mix well.

3. In a separate bowl, combine the alaria, cucumbers, and watercress. Pour the dressing over the salad, toss, and serve.

BEET SALAD

SERVINGS: 4 to 6

I pound beets

2 tablespoons mustard

3 tablespoons balsamic vinegar

$1/_4$ cup olive oil

I Bermuda onion, diced

Sea salt to taste

Black pepper to taste

1. In a 4½-quart saucepan, cover the beets with water and bring to a boil. Lower the heat to medium, cover, and cook for approximately 1 hour, or until tender through the middle. Drain and cool. Slice the beets and place them in a mixing bowl.

2. In another mixing bowl, combine the mustard, balsamic vinegar, olive oil, Bermuda onion, sea salt, and pepper. Mix well and pour over the beets. Marinate for several hours or overnight. Serve at room temperature.

DAIKON RADISH SALAD

SERVINGS: 4 to 6

1 cup grated daikon radish	½ teaspoon sea salt
½ cup thinly sliced scallions	Juice of 1 lemon
1 cup grated carrot	

1. In a mixing bowl, combine the daikon radish, scallions, carrot, sea salt, and lemon juice.

2. Mix well and serve.

PRESSED CUCUMBER SALAD

SERVINGS: 4 to 6

4 cucumbers, peeled and sliced	1 teaspoon toasted sesame oil
1 teaspoon sea salt	1 teaspoon brown rice vinegar
1 teaspoon tamari	3 tablespoons toasted sesame seeds

1. Place cucumbers and sea salt in a pickle press or bowl with a weight on top. Press for 1 hour or more. Drain the liquid and rinse off the sea salt.

2. Place the cucumbers in a mixing bowl. Add the tamari, toasted sesame oil, and brown rice vinegar. Garnish with the toasted sesame seeds and serve.

RUTABAGA PICKLES

SERVINGS: 4 to 6

2 cups thinly sliced rutabaga   2 cups tamari

2 cups water

1. Place sliced rutabaga in a pickle press or bowl. In a mixing bowl, combine the water and tamari. Mix well. Cover rutabaga with mixture. Put top on pickle press, or place a weight on top of rutabaga in bowl.

2. Press rutabaga for at least 4 hours, but ideally overnight. Serve.

MISO DRESSING

SERVINGS: 2 to 4

3 tablespoons white miso   1 clove garlic, minced

1 tablespoon apple cider vinegar   1 teaspoon freshly grated ginger

1 teaspoon olive oil

1. In a mixing bowl, combine the white miso, apple cider vinegar, olive oil, and garlic. Mix well.

MISO TAHINI SAUCE

SERVINGS: 2 to 4

$1/2$ cup white miso   Juice of 1 lemon

3 tablespoons tahini

1. In a $1^{1}/_{2}$-quart saucepan over low heat, combine the white miso, tahini, and lemon juice. Stir well, adding enough water to make a sauce. Simmer for 10 minutes.

MUSTARD DRESSING

SERVINGS: 2 to 4

Juice of 2 lemons

4 tablespoons tamari

2 teaspoons mustard

2 tablespoons tahini

1. In a mixing bowl, combine the lemon juice, tamari, mustard, and tahini. Mix well.

SCALLION AND PARSLEY DRESSING

SERVINGS: 2 to 4

$1/4$ cup finely sliced scallions

1 tablespoon finely chopped fresh parsley

1 teaspoon olive oil

1 tablespoon lemon juice

1 tablespoon apple cider vinegar

Pinch of sea salt

Enough water for desired consistency

1. Place the scallions, parsley, olive oil, lemon juice, apple cider vinegar, sea salt, and water in a jar. Cover and shake until blended.

TOFU SALAD DRESSING

SERVINGS: 2 to 4

$1/2$ teaspoon freshly grated ginger

16 ounces soft tofu

$1/4$ cup water

2 tablespoons white miso

2 tablespoons apple cider vinegar

1. In a blender, combine the ginger, tofu, water, white miso, and apple cider vinegar. Blend thoroughly.

PURE LEMON
SALAD DRESSING

SERVINGS: 2 to 4

Juice from 3 lemons

$^1/_2$ cup tamari

1. In a mixing bowl, combine the lemon juice and tamari. Mix well.

SESAME LEMON
SALAD DRESSING

SERVINGS: 2 to 4

2 tablespoons toasted sesame oil

3 tablespoons lemon juice

2 tablespoons tamari

$^1/_2$ cup water

1. Place the toasted sesame oil, lemon juice, tamari, and water in a jar. Cover and shake until blended.

VINAIGRETTE

SERVINGS: 2 to 4

2 tablespoons minced onion

1 tablespoon mustard

3 tablespoons apple cider vinegar

$^1/_2$ tablespoon olive oil

1 teaspoon tamari

1. Place the onion, mustard, apple cider vinegar, olive oil, and tamari in a jar. Cover and shake until blended.

SESAME SEED
AND SCALLION CONDIMENT

SERVINGS: 2 to 4

I tablespoon olive oil	I cup sliced scallion
I cup diced onion	I tablespoon gluten- free miso
I cup diced red pepper	I cup sesame seeds

1. In a large skillet, sauté the onion, red pepper, and scallion in the olive oil for 5 minutes, or until tender.

2. Add the miso and sauté for 3 minutes. Add the sesame seeds, toss, and use as a condiment on grains.

SESAME SEED
AND SEAWEED CONDIMENT

SERVINGS: 2 to 4

I part dulse seaweed	10 parts sesame seeds, rinsed

1. Preheat oven to 350°F.

2. Place the dulse seaweed on a baking sheet and dry roast in oven for 15 minutes, or until crispy.

3. In a large skillet over low heat, dry roast the sesame seeds until they begin to pop, stirring constantly to avoid burning.

4. Crush the seaweed and seeds together in a suribachi, or process them in a blender.

BEANS

ADUKI BEANS
WITH SQUASH AND KELP

SERVINGS: 4 to 6

$^1/_2$ cup aduki beans,
rinsed and soaked overnight

2 strips kelp

1 winter squash, cubed

Tamari to taste

1. In a $4^1/_2$-quart saucepan, combine the aduki beans, kelp, and squash. Cover with water and bring to a boil. Cook for 20 minutes. Lower the heat to simmer, cover, and cook for $1^1/_2$ hours, or until beans are soft.

2. Add the tamari. Cover, simmer for 15 minutes, and serve.

BLACK BEAN CHILI

SERVINGS: 4 to 6

2 cups dried black beans,
soaked overnight

1 strip kelp

1 large onion, diced

1 large carrot, diced

1 green bell pepper, cubed

2 cloves garlic, thinly sliced

1 tablespoon chili powder

2 tablespoons dark gluten-free miso,
or to taste

1. In a $4^1/_2$-quart saucepan, combine the black beans and kelp, cover with water, and bring to a boil. Lower the heat to simmer, cover, and cook for $1^1/_2$ hours, or until beans are tender.

2. Add the onion, carrot, bell pepper, garlic, and chili powder. Simmer for 20 minutes. Add the miso and continue to simmer for 10 minutes.

MACARONI AND BEAN SALAD

SERVINGS: 4 to 6

3 cups cooked gluten-free macaroni

1 $^1/_2$ cups cooked kidney beans

4 scallions, chopped

2 celery stalks, chopped

Handful of finely chopped
fresh parsley

6 tablespoons lemon juice

4 tablespoons tamari

2 teaspoons mustard

2 tablespoons tahini

6 tablespoons water

1. In a large salad bowl, combine the macaroni, kidney beans, scallions, celery, and parsley. Toss well.

2. In a small jar, combine the lemon juice, tamari, mustard, tahini, and water. Cover and shake until blended. Pour over the macaroni and bean salad. Toss well and allow it to sit for at least 15 minutes before serving.

MARINATED CHICKPEA SALAD

SERVINGS: 4 to 6

3 cups cooked garbanzo beans

2 tablespoons olive oil

3 tablespoons apple cider vinegar

Pinch sea salt

6 red radishes, diced

1 small cucumber, peeled and diced

2 stalks celery

$^1/_2$ cup thinly sliced watercress

1 tablespoon fresh parsley

1 teaspoon fresh dill

1. In a large mixing bowl, combine the garbanzo beans, olive oil, apple cider vinegar, and sea salt. Cover and allow the beans to marinate for at least 1 hour. You can also leave them in the refrigerator overnight.

2. Add the radishes, cucumber, celery, watercress, parsley, and dill. Mix well and allow to chill before serving.

SCRAMBLED TOFU

SERVINGS: 2 to 4

I tablespoon sesame oil

I onion, diced

I carrot, chopped

$^1/_2$ stalk celery, chopped

14-ounce container soft tofu

I teaspoon cumin

I teaspoon turmeric

$^1/_4$ teaspoon black pepper

$^1/_2$ teaspoon tamari

1. In a large skillet, sauté the onion, carrot, and celery in the sesame oil for 3 minutes.

2. Crumble the tofu into the skillet. Add the cumin, turmeric, pepper, and tamari. Cover and cook for 10 minutes, stirring frequently, and serve.

MAKE-YOUR-OWN HUMMUS

SERVINGS: 2 to 4

3 cups cooked garbanzo beans

I cup tahini

$^1/_4$ cup lemon juice

3 cloves garlic, minced

$^1/_2$ teaspoon white pepper

I teaspoon sea salt

1. In a large mixing bowl, combine the garbanzo beans, tahini, and lemon juice. Purée, adding water as needed to make the texture creamy.

2. Add the garlic, pepper, and sea salt. Mix well and allow to chill before serving.

SWEET PINTO BEANS

SERVINGS: 2 to 4

2 cups pinto beans,
soaked overnight

1 strip kombu

$^3/_4$ cup dark miso

$^1/_4$ cup unsweetened apple butter

1 tablespoon mustard

1. Preheat oven to 350°F.

2. In a $4^1/_2$-quart saucepan, combine the pinto beans and kombu, cover with water, and bring to a boil. Lower the heat to simmer, cover, and cook for $1^1/_2$ hours, or until beans are tender.

3. In a mixing bowl, combine the miso, apple butter, and mustard. Mix well. (Proportions of miso and apple butter may be adjusted depending on whether you would like a sweeter or more savory dish.)

4. In a large glass baking dish, combine the cooked pinto beans and miso mixture. Bake for at least 30 minutes.

FISH

BAKED WHITEFISH

SERVINGS: 2 to 4

Juice of 1 lemon	$^1/_2$ cup fresh basil
4 tablespoons olive oil	1 tablespoons tamari
$^1/_2$ cup fresh dill	2 pounds whitefish

1. Preheat oven to 375°F.

2. In a small mixing bowl, combine the lemon juice, olive oil, dill, basil, and tamari. Mix well.

3. Place the fish in a large baking dish. Pour the lemon juice mixture on top of the fish. Bake for 20 minutes, or until fish is completely cooked.

WHITEFISH CIOPPINO

SERVINGS: 4 to 6

2 pounds of whitefish	1 teaspoon sea salt
$^1/_2$ cup diced yellow onion	$^1/_2$ teaspoon black pepper
$^1/_2$ cup sliced leeks	2 tablespoons olive oil
3 carrots, sliced	4 cups water
2 cups sliced button mushrooms	1 cup chopped fresh basil
4 cloves garlic, minced	

1. In a 6-quart stockpot, sauté the onion, leeks, carrots, mushrooms, garlic, sea salt, and pepper in the olive oil until vegetables are soft. Add the water, cover, and simmer for approximately 40 minutes.

2. Add the fish, cover, and simmer for ten minutes, or until fish is completely cooked. Garnish with the basil and serve.

FAVORITE FISH DISH

SERVINGS: 2 to 4

Olive oil to taste, divided

2 onions, sliced

2 cloves garlic, thinly sliced

3 cups chopped Chinese cabbage or spinach

1 leek, sliced

1 cup button mushrooms, stems removed, sliced

2 pounds whitefish

1 teaspoon dill

1 teaspoon basil

Lemon juice to taste

Tamari to taste

Fresh parsley, chopped, to taste

1. In a large skillet, sauté the onions, garlic, Chinese cabbage, leek, and mushrooms in the olive oil for 10 minutes, or until soft. Place whitefish on top. Season with the dill and basil.

2. In a mixing bowl, combine the lemon juice, tamari, and olive oil. Mix well and pour over the entire dish. Cover and simmer until fish is done. Garnish with parsley and serve.

WHITEFISH SALAD

SERVINGS: 2 to 4

1 pound whitefish, steamed

1 cup diced celery

1 cup thinly sliced scallions

1 tablespoon olive oil

1 teaspoon apple cider vinegar

1 teaspoon tamari

1. With a fork or masher, lightly mash the steamed whitefish.

2. In a large mixing bowl, combine the mashed whitefish, celery, scallions, olive oil, apple cider vinegar, and tamari. Mix well. Serve on top of salad or enjoy with gluten-free crackers.

WEEKLY MENU PLAN

The following menu plan will help you balance your daily meals. Use the plan as a guide until you are comfortable putting your own meal plans together. Remember to enjoy the process! In time, you will feel confident enough to allow your intuition to lead you.

MONDAY, DAY ONE

Breakfast:

Simple Miso Soup

Oatmeal

Boiled Kale with Sesame
Lemon Salad Dressing

Lunch:

Simple Brown Rice

Indian Vegetable Curry

Pressed Cucumber Salad

Dinner:

Squash Soup

Simple Brown Rice with Sesame Seed and Seaweed Condiment

Black Bean Chili

Sautéed Bok Choy with Miso Dressing

TUESDAY, DAY TWO

Breakfast:

Simple Miso Soup

Simple Brown Rice

Scrambled Tofu

Sautéed Bok Choy
with Miso Dressing

Tea

Lunch:

Greek Spirals

Mixed Greens

Dinner:

Shiitake Mushroom and Quinoa Soup

Sweet Pinto Beans

Simple Brown Rice with Sesame Seed and Scallion Condiment

Chinese Vegetables

WEDNESDAY, DAY THREE

Breakfast:

Simple Miso Soup

Oatmeal

Boiled Kale with Pure
Lemon Salad Dressing

Lunch:

Buckwheat and Macaroni

Boiled Collard Greens
with Vinaigrette

Daikon Radish Salad

Dinner:

Whitefish Cioppino

Simple Brown Rice with Sesame Seed and Scallion Condiment

Sautéed Leafy Greens with your choice of dressing

Rutabaga Pickles

THURSDAY, DAY FOUR

Breakfast:

Simple Miso Soup

Oatmeal

Boiled Broccoli with Pure
Lemon Salad Dressing

Lunch:

Noodles with Sauce

Ratatouille

Cucumber, Alaria,
and Watercress Salad

Dinner:

Minestrone Soup

Quinoa Salad

Favorite Fish Dish

Luscious Leeks

Boiled Kale with Tofu Salad Dressing

FRIDAY, DAY FIVE

Breakfast:

Simple Miso Soup

Oatmeal

Sautéed Leafy Greens
with your choice of dressing

Lunch:

Simple Brown Rice

Marinated Chickpea Salad

Sautéed Broccoli

Dinner:

Red Lentil Soup

Indian Vegetable Curry

Simple Brown Rice

Pressed Cucumber Salad

Sautéed Leafy Greens

SATURDAY, DAY SIX

Breakfast:

Simple Miso Soup

Simple Brown Rice

Sautéed Collard Greens
with your choice of dressing

Lunch:

Noodles with Sauce

Beet Salad

Mixed Greens

Dinner:

Curried Cauliflower Soup

Japanese Fried Rice

Baked Root Stew

Boiled Leafy Greens with Scallion and Parsley Dressing

SUNDAY, DAY SEVEN

Breakfast:

Simple Miso Soup

Oatmeal

Boiled Leafy Greens
with your choice of dressing

Lunch:

Buckwheat and Macaroni

Cucumber, Alaria,
and Watercress Salad

Rutabaga and Dill

Dinner:

Dried Mushroom and Spinach Soup

Japanese Fried Rice

Boiled Kale with Mustard Dressing

Whitefish Salad

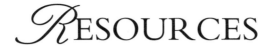

ℛESOURCES

Below you will find contact information for a number of different people and institutions that provide the various kinds of health and healing services described in this book.

DIET, EXERCISE, AND LIFESTYLE

La Ferme du Bois-le-Comte
Bois-le-Comte 1
6823 Villers-devant-Orval
Orval, Belgium
+32 61 32 99 20
https://boislecomte.be/
La Ferme du Bois-le-Comte provides a wide range of programs in natural healing and lifestyle, yoga, macrobiotics, shiatsu, five rhythms dance, shamanism, agriculture, permaculture, and many other approaches to health.

Instituto Macrobiótico de Portugal
Rua Anchieta, 5 - 2º Esq.
1200–023 Lisboa
+351 22 324 22 90
info@institutomacrobiotico.com
www.institutomacrobiotico.com/en

Instituto Macrobiótico de Portugal offers courses in all facets of macrobiotic education, healing, and philosophy. Founded in 1985 and directed by Francisco Varatojo, the center also provides personal counseling and individual lifestyle approaches to health and healing.

The Kushi Instsitute of Europe
Weteringschans 65
1017 RX Amsterdam, NL
+31 (0)20 625 75 13
info@macrobiotics.nl
www.macrobiotics.nl
The Kushi Institute of Europe (Amsterdam) was established in 1975 and has been providing a wide array of courses in macrobiotic education, philosophy, natural lifestyle, healing, and cooking. The center also provides a lunch and take-out meal service.

Macrobiotics America
1735 Robinson St., #1874
Oroville, CA 95965-9998
(530) 521-0236
(530) 282-3518
info@macroamerica.com
www.macroamerica.com
Macrobiotics America is directed by
David and Cynthia Briscoe, teachers
and counselors of macrobiotic educa-
tion, lifestyle, philosophy, and cooking.
With more than thirty years experi-
ence, they provide personal counseling
in the macrobiotic lifestyle, philosophy,
and approach to health and healing.

Macrobiotics Today
George Oshawa Macrobiotic
Foundation
1277 Marin Avenue
Chico, CA 95928
(530) 566-9765
gomf@ohsawamacrobiotics.com
www.ohsawamacrobiotics.com/ma
crobiotics-today
Macrobiotics Today is a magazine
that provides information on macrobi-
otic teachings and services, including
cooking classes and counseling in the
macrobiotic way of life in communities
throughout the country.

Dr. McDougall's Health
& Medical Center
P.O. Box 14039
Santa Rosa, CA 95402
(800) 941-7111
(707) 538-8609
office@drmcdougall.com

www.drmcdougall.com
Dr. McDougall's Health & Medical
Center provides doctor-supervised live-
in programs based on the McDougall
approach to diet and exercise for the
treatment of a wide variety of illnesses.

The Pritikin Longevity Center
and Spa
8755 NW 36th Street
Miami, Florida 33178
(888) 254-1462
(305) 935-7131
www.pritikin.com
The Pritikin Longevity Center and
Spa provides educational programs
in the scientifically based Pritikin
diet, exercise, and lifestyle. It offers
accommodations and doctor-supervised
medical care to its guests.

The Strengthening Health Institute
1940 South 10th Street
Philadelphia, PA 19148
(215) 238-9212
info.strengthenhealth@gmail.com
www.strengthenhealth.org
The Strengthening Health Institute,
directed by long-time macrobiotic
teacher and counselor Denny Wax-
man, provides classes in macrobiotic
philosophy, lifestyle, and cooking.
Waxman also provides counseling
services in the use of macrobiotics
to improve health and healing.

Virginia Harper
615-646-2841
info@youcanhealyou.com

www.youcanhealyou.com
Virginia Harper, of Nashville, Tennessee, provides education and guidance in the use of a macrobiotic diet and lifestyle to control symptoms of Crohn's disease and other inflammatory bowel disorders.

FOOD

Eden Foods
701 Tecumseh Road
Clinton, Michigan 49236
(888) 424-3336
info@edenfoods.com
www.edenfoods.com
Established in the late 1960s, Eden Foods specializes in providing the highest quality natural, organic, and macrobiotic foods. Eden foods prides itself on offering foods that are non-GMO, non-irradiated, and packaged i n containers that are free of bisphenol-A and other toxic substances.

Gold Mine Natural Food Co.
13200 Danielson Street, Suite A-1
Poway, CA 92064
(800) 475-3663
customerservice@goldminenatural-foods.com
www.goldminenaturalfoods.com
Started in 1985, Gold Mine Natural Food Co. is a mail-order grocer that provides a vast array of natural and organic foods and macrobiotic staples. Located in Southern California, Gold Mine offers everything from beans, grains, pastas, sea vegetables, sauerkraut and

condiments, beverages, cookware, personal care, books, and much more.

Jaffe Bro. Natural Foods
Organic Fruits and Nuts
28560 Lilac Road
Valley Center, CA 92032
(760) 749-1133
jaffebros@att.net
www.organicfruitsandnuts.com
Located in Southern California, Jaffe Bro. Natural Foods is a mail-order grocer that sells a wide assortment of organic fruits, nuts, grains, natural sweeteners, flours and baking products, olives, sauerkraut, dehydrated vegetables, and many other staples.

Maine Seaweed
P.O. Box 57
Steuben, ME 04680
(207) 546-2875
info@theseaweedman.com
http://theseaweedman.com
One of the pioneers of the macrobiotic and natural foods movement, Larch Hanson has been harvesting sea vegetables in off the coast of Maine for four decades. Maine Seaweed is a mail-order supply business that provides a wide array of seaweeds, as well as recipes, videos, a regular blog, and nutritional information on the company's seaweed products.

Natural Lifestyle
16 Lookout Drive
Asheville, NC 28804
(800) 752-2775

order@natural-lifestyle.com
www.natural-lifestyle.com
*Natural Lifestyle is a mail-order
natural and organic foods grocer that
sells a wide assortment of beans, nuts,
grains, fruit, teas, miso and other soybean products, cookware, supplements,
and books on health and well-being.*

HEALTH AND HEALING

Caldwell Esselstyn, MD
Cleveland Clinic Wellness Institute
1950 Richmond Road
Lyndhurst, Ohio 44124
(216) 448-8556
EssyProgram@ccf.org
www.dresselstyn.com/site/
*Based on his bestselling book Prevent
and Reverse Heart Disease: The Revolutionary, Scientifically Proven, Nutrition-Based Cure, Dr. Caldwell Esselstyn's
website provides articles, DVDs, and
videos for overcoming heart disease
and other cardiovascular illnesses
through the use of a plant-based diet.*

Cleveland Clinic
www.clevelandclinic.org
*The Cleveland Clinic website provides
a vast medical library that can be
accessed for free.*

Derek Henry
http://healingthebody.ca
*Derek Henry created the online program
"Healing the Body" to empower people
in their own health transformations.
With a large database of helpful articles*

*on nutrition, mindset, therapies, and
lifestyle choices, it is a premier resource
for people hoping to help themselves.*

Institute of Integrative Nutrition
www.integrativenutrition.com
*The largest online nutrition school, the
Institute of Integrative Nutrition seeks
to start a health revolution by offering
training courses to people around the
world who wish to become health coaches.*

Jeanette Bronée
Path for Life
http://pathforlife.com
*Jeanette Bronée is an author, speaker,
and creator of the self-nourishment
practice "Path for Life," which focuses
on the power of healing through
nutrition and lifestyle.*

Mayo Clinic
www.mayoclinic.org
*The Mayo Clinic website provides a
wealth of free information on illnesses
of all types. It also offers details on the
clinic's vast medical services.*

PubMed
www.pubmed.gov
*PubMed is the online US National
Library of Medicine for the National
Institutes of Health. It offers peer-
reviewed scientific studies in all areas
of health and illness.*

**T. Colin Campbell Center for
Nutrition Studies**
P.O. Box 7256

Ithaca, NY 14851
(607) 319-0287
http://nutritionstudies.org
*Created to advocate the research of
Dr. T. Colin Campbell, coauthor of the
landmark book* The China Study, *the T.
Colin Campbell Center for Nutritional
Studies offers an array of online articles
and educational programs regarding
the application of a plant-based diet in
the prevention of serious illness and
the restoration of health.*

WebMd

www.webmd.com
*WebMd offers medical and health
information on individual illnesses,
drugs and supplements, diet, nutrition, pregnancy, and family issues.*

INTERCESSORY PRAYER

Beliefnet

www.beliefnet.com
*This website offers an array of groups
that can be contacted online for intercessory prayer.*

Padmasambhava Buddhist Center Prayer Requests

Padma Samye Ling
618 Buddha Highway
Sidney Center, NY 13839
(607) 865-8068
jowozegyal@catskill.net
www.padmasambhava.org/prayer-
req.html
This Buddhist meditation and study

*center accepts prayer requests which
they fulfill in daily ceremonies.*

Catholic Prayer Requests

www.catholicprayerrequests.com
*Roman Catholic nuns and priests
take prayer requests from people of all
faiths through this website and pray
for them daily.*

Order of Carmelites

Carmelite vocation office
Carith House
5498 S. Kimbark Ave.
Chicago, IL 60615-5208
(773) 322-1222
carmelites@carmelites.net
www.carmelites.net
*The Carmelites are a Roman Catholic
order that prays on behalf of others.*

Discalced Carmelite Nuns of the Carmel of Saint Joseph

http://www.stlouiscarmel.com/ab
out-us-3/
*The Discalced Carmelite Nuns of
the Carmel of Saint Joseph pray for
individuals and the world. They may
be contacted with prayer requests
through their website.*

Tehilim Hotline

(888) 448-3445
(718) 851-2365
info@tehilimhotline.org
www.tehilimhotline.org
*This hotline offers twenty-hour service
to Jews seeking help through the power
of prayer.*

Virtual Jerusalem
www.virtualjerusalem.com
*Virtual Jerusalem is a Jewish online
magazine. It takes prayer requests and
will place written requests in the Wailing Wall in Jerusalem.*

**PHYSICAL THERAPY AND
HEALING TOUCH**

**American Academy of Medical
Acupressure**
2512 Artesia Blvd, Ste 200
Redondo Beach, CA 90278
(310) 379-8261
info@medicalacupuncture.org
www.medicalacupuncture.org
*Acupressure is based on the same princi-
ples as acupuncture, only this technique
uses fingers and hands to stimulate the
flow of life energy along the fourteen
pathways known in Chinese medicine
as meridians and restore health.*

**American Society for the
Alexander Technique**
11 West Monument Avenue,
Suite 510
Dayton, OH 45402-1233
(937) 586-3732
(800) 473-0620
www.amsatonline.org/teachers
*The Alexander technique focuses
primarily on correcting posture and
the many disorders that can arise from
distortions in posture. Practitioners
use hands and corrective exercises to
correct imbalances in posture and
encourage harmony in the body.*

**The Biodynamic Craniosacral Therapy
Association of North America**
www.craniosacraltherapy.org
*Craniosacral release involves balancing
the craniosacral system, which includes
the skull, spinal column, sacrum, and
all nerves and tissues housed within
these structures. Through very gentle
manipulation of the body, the practitioner releases blocks within the craniosacral system to release trauma, old
wounds, and sources of illness.*

Emotional Freedom Technique (EFT)
www.emofree.com
*Sometimes called "tapping," Emotional
Freedom Technique, or EFT, is a version
of acupuncture without the use of needles.
Instead, subjects tap meridian points on
their bodies with their fingertips.*

Ericksonian Hypnotherapy
2632 E Thomas Road, Suite 200
Phoenix, AZ 85016
(602) 956-6196
(877) 212-6678
support@erickson-foundation.org
www.erickson-foundation.org
*Hypnosis is a therapeutic tool to help
people access their inner resources to
heal and grow. It is not stage hypnosis
that purports to makes us forget who
we are. Rather, it is a way to bypass
the inner critic and access the inner
coach, that aspect of self that can guide
us to happiness and success.*

Jin Shin Jyutsu
www.jsjinc.net

Jin Shin Jyutsu is based on the theory that pathways of life energy, known as flows, traverse the body and bring life force to organs, systems, and tissues. This physio-philosophy aims to unblock this life energy and bring harmony to the body.

Shiatsu

www.takingcharge.csh.umn.edu/explore-healing-practices/shiatsu
Shiatsu is the Japanese form of acupressure. Like acupressure, it has been practiced for thousands of years. Practitioners use finger pressure to stimulate acupuncture points and increase the flow of energy along meridian lines, thereby promoting healing in organs and bodily systems. To learn more about shiatsu and find a practitioner, visit the website of the University of Minnesota's Center for Spirituality & Healing.

Ohashiatsu

www.ohashi.com
Ohashiatsu is a form of shiatsu, the Japanese form of acupressure. It combines shiatsu, exercise, meditation, and ancient diagnostic techniques to recognize imbalances, boost life energy along meridians, restore harmony to organs and bodily systems, and relieve tension.

Reflexology

https://www.takingcharge.csh.umn.edu/explore-healing-practices/reflexology
*Reflexology is a form of acupressure that uses finger pressure to stimulate certain points on the feet that corre-*spond to specific organs and systems, thus increasing life force to these parts of the body and relieving tension. To learn more about reflexology and find a practitioner, visit the website of the University of Minnesota's Center for Spirituality & Healing.*

Reiki

http://reiki-directory.com
Reiki is a Tibetan form of laying on of hands. Practitioners channel life energy into their clients' bodies by placing their hands over specific parts of the body. This increase in life energy is meant to support organ function, elevate mood, and relieve tension. There are numerous online directories through which to find Reiki practitioners around the world.

Swedish Massage

http://www.byregion.net/main-search/search/WorldHealers/bodyworkers/Swedish%20Massage
Swedish massage is often referred to as deep tissue massage because practitioners often work the muscles extensively. They also use gentle rubbing and finger techniques to relieve tension and take muscles out of spasm. Swedish massage is among the oldest forms of massage practiced in the West. Practitioners of Swedish massage may be found in virtually every major city in the world.

Worldwide Directory of Healing Touch Practitioners

http://htpractitioner.com/component/comprofiler/userslist
Healing touch is a form of laying on of hands. Practitioners either place their hands gently on their subjects' bodies or just above them, working on what they call the "energy body," or "aura," and attempting to relieve pain and reduce stress levels.

American Dance Therapy Association
10632 Little Patuxent Parkway, Suite 108
Columbia, MD 21044
(410) 997-4040
info@adta.org
https://adta.org
Dance and movement therapies are designed to help people experience, express, and release painful feelings and heal old wounds and traumas, which lead to ill health. Among the most widely practiced dance and move-ment therapies are yoga, the five rhythms, and the Feldenkrais method.

VOLUNTEERING

Experience Corps
http://www.aarp.org/experience-corps/
Experience Corps is an AARP Foundation literacy program that pairs volunteer tutors fifty years of age or older with fourth-graders who are struggling with reading skills to improve the literacy of students in their own communities.

Volunteer Match
www.volunteermatch.org
Volunteer Match connects people who would like to volunteer with good causes that could benefit from their help. It can put people in touch with the non-profit organizations that are most compatible with their goals.

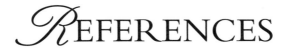

REFERENCES

Step One

Goleman, Daniel. "Seeking Out Small Pleasures Keeps Immune System Strong." *New York Times* 11 May 1994. Accessed 12 Mar. 2015. http://www.nytimes.com/1994/05/11/garden/seeking-out-small-pleasures-keeps-immune-system-strong.html

Irwin, Michael. "Plasma cortisol and natural killer cell activity during bereavement." *Biological Psychiatry* 24.2 (1988): 173–178. Print.

Kushi, Michio, with Alex Jack. *The Cancer Prevention Diet.* New York: St. Martin's Press, 1993. Print.

McKenna, Marlene, with Tom Monte. *When Hope Never Dies.* New York: Kensington Books, 2000. Print.

Reiche, Edna Maria, et al. "Stress, depression, the immune system, and cancer." *The Lancet Oncology* 5.10 (2004): 617–625. Print.

Schleifer, Steven, et al. "Suppression of Lymphocyte stimulation following bereavement." *Journal of the American Medical Association* 250.3 (1983): 374–377. Print.

Step Two

Campbell, T. Colin. *The China Study: The Most Comprehensive Study of Nutrition Ever Conducted.* Dallas: BenBella Books, 2005. Print.

Dossey, Larry. *Space, Time, and Medicine.* Boston: Shambhala, 1982. Print.

Esselstyn, Caldwell B. *Prevent and Reverse Heart Disease: The Revolutionary Scientifically Proven, Nutrition-Based Cure.* New York: Penguin Group, 2007. Print.

Harper, Virginia, with Tom Monte. *Controlling Crohn's Disease: The Natural Way.* New York: Kensington Publishers, 2002. Print.

Laudenslager, ML, Ryan, SM, et al. "Coping and immunosuppression:

inescapable but not escapable school suppresses lymphocyte proliferation." *Science* 221.4610 (1983): 568–570. Print.

McDougall, John, and Mary McDougall. *The Starch Solution. Eat the Foods You Love, Regain Your Health, and Lose the Weight for Good!* Emmaus, PA: Rodale Press, 2012. Print.

Monte, Tom, with Ilene Pritikin. *Pritikin: The Man Who Healed America's Heart.* Emmaus, PA: Rodale Press, 1988. Print.

New York-Presbyterian Hospital. "Patient Education And Empowerment Can Improve Health Outcomes For Diabetes Patients." *New York-Presbyterian Hospital* 8 August 2014. Accessed 15 Jan. 2015. http://www.nyp.org/news/Patient-Education-Empowerment-Improve-Health-Outcomes-Diabetes

Ornish, Dean, et al. "Can lifestyle changes reverse coronary heart disease? The Lifestyle Heart Trial." *The Lancet* 336.8715 (1990): 624—626. Print.

Sieber, William J., Rodin, Judith, et al. "Modulatoin of human natural killer cell activity by exposure to uncontrollable stress. Brain, Behavior, and Immunity. June 1992; 6(2): 141–156. Print.

Siegel, Bernie. *Love, Medicine, and Miracles.* New York: HarperCollins, 1986. Print.

Step Three

Abdulla, M., Gruber, P. "Role of diet modification in cancer prevention." *Biofactors* 12.1–4 (2000): 45–51. Print.

Adam, Tanja C., and Elissa S. Eppel. "Stress, eating and reward system." *Physiology and Behavior* 91.4 (2007): 449–458. Print.

Ames, B.N. "Micronutrients prevent cancer and delay aging." *Toxicology Letters* 102–103 (1998): 5–18. Print.

Ames, B.N. "Micronutrients prevent cancer and delay aging." *Toxicology* 102–103 (1998): 5–18. Print.

Anand, Preetha, et al. "Cancer is a Preventable Disease that Requires Major Lifestyle Changes." *Pharmaceutical Research* 25.9 (2008): 2097–2116. Print.

Augustin, L.S.A., et al. "Dietary glycemic index and glycemic load, and breast cancer risk: a case-controlled study." *Annals of Oncology* 12.11 (2001): 1533–1538. Print.

Bala, D.V., Patel, D.D., et al. "Role of Dietary Intake and Biomarkers in Risk of Breast Cancer: A Case Control Study." *Asian Pacific Journal of Cancer Prevention* 2.2 (2001): 123–130. Print.

Barnard, R.J., et al. "Prostate cancer: Another aspect of the insulin-resistance syndrome?" *Obesity Reviews* 3.4 (2002): 3003–3008. Print.

Barnard, R.J., et al. "Response of non-insulin-dependent diabetic patients to an intensive program of diet and exercise." *Diabetes Care* 5.4 (1982): 370–374. Print.

Boyd, M.F., Stone, J., et al. "Dietary fat and breast cancer risk revisited: a meta analysis of the published literature." *British Journal of Cancer* 89.9 (2003): 1672–1685. Print.

Bray, George A., Lovejoy, Jennifer C., et al. "The Influence of Different Fats and Fatty Acids on Obesity, Insulin Resistance, and Inflammation." *Journal of Nutrition* 132.9 (2002): 2488–2491. Print.

Broekmans, W.M., et al. "Fruits and vegetables increase plasma carotenoids and vitamins and decrease homocysteine in humans." *Journal of Nutrition* 130.6 (2000): 1578–1583. Print.

Calle, Eugenia E., Rodriguez, C., et al. "Overweight, Obesity, and Mortality from Cancer in a Prospectively Studied Cohort of U.S. Adults." *New England Journal of Medicine* 348 (2003): 1625–1638. Print.

Campbell, T. Colin. *The China Study: The Most Comprehensive Study of Nutrition Ever Conducted.* Dallas: BenBella Books, 2005. Print.

Carey, Benedict, "Genes as Mirrors of Life Experiences." *New York Times* 8 Nov. 2010. Accessed 10 Mar. 2015.
http://www.nytimes.com/2010/11/09/health/09brain.html

Carter, J.P., et al., "Hypothesis: Dietary Management May improve Survival from Nutritionally Linked Cancers Based on Analysis of Representative Cases." *Journal of the American College of Nutrition* 12.3 (1993): 209–226. Print.

Cavallo, M.G., et al. "Cell-mediated immune response to beta-casein in recent-onset insulin-dependent diabetes: implications for disease pathogenesis." *The Lancet* 348.9032 (1996): 926–928. Print.

Cho, Eunyoung, et al. "Premenopausal Fat Intake and Risk of Breast Cancer." *Journal of the National Cancer Institute* 95.14 (2003): 1079–1085. Print.

Cho, Eunyoung, et al. "Red Meat Intake and Breast Cancer among Premenopausal Women." *Archives of Internal Medicine* 166.20 (2006): 2253–2259. Print.

Craft, Susanne. "Insulin resistance syndrome and Alzheimer's disease: Age- and obesity-related effect on memory, amyloid, and inflammation." *Neurobiology of Aging* 26.1 (2005): 65–69. Print.

Cramer, D.W., Harlow, B.L., and Willet, W.C. "Galactose consumption and metabolism in relation to risk of ovarian cancer." *The Lancet* 2.8654 (1989): 66–71. Print.

De Marzo, A.M., DeWeese, T.L., et al. "Pathological and molecular mechanisms of prostate carcinogenesis: implications for diagnosis, detection, prevention, and treatment." *Journal of Cell Biochemistry* 91.3 (2004): 459–477. Print.

De Marzo, A.M., et al. "Human prostate cancer precursors and pathobiology." *Journal of Urology* 62.5 Suppl 1 (2003): 55–62. Print.

DeNoon, Daniel J. "Some Herbs May Fight Cancer." *WebMD* 28 Oct. 2003. Accessed 21 Mar. 2015. http://www.webmd.com/cancer/news/20031028/some-herbs-may-fight-cancer#1

Di Fiore, Nancy. "Diet May Help Prevent Alzheimer's Disease." *Rush University Medical Center* Accessed 20 April 2016. https://www.rush.edu/news/diet-may-help-prevent-alzheimers

Duke University Medical Center. "Epigenetics Means What we Eat, How We Live and Love, Alters How Our Genes Behave." *Science Daily* 27 October 2005. Accessed 26 Jan. 2015. https://www.sciencedaily.com/releases/2005/10/051026090636.htm

Fleshner, N.E., Klotz, L.H. "Diet, androgens oxidative stress and prostate cancer susceptibility." Journal of Cancer Metastasis Reviews 17.4 (1998–1999): 325–330. Print.

Fred Hutchinson Cancer Research Center. "Move over tomatoes! All vegetables—especially the cruciferous kind—may prevent prostate cancer." *Fred Hutchinson Cancer Research Center* 4 January 2000. Accessed 15 Nov. 2015. https://www.fredhutch.org/en/news/releases/2000/01/Veggiesprostat.html

Galli, R.L., et al. "Fruit polyphenolics and brain aging: nutritional intervention targeting age-related neuronal and behavioral benefits." *Annals of New York Academy of Sciences* 959 (2002): 128–132. Print.

Ganmaa, D., et al. "Incidence and mortality of testicular cancer and prostatic cancers in relation to world dietary practices." *International Journal of Cancer* 98.2 (2002): 262–267. Print.

Gao, X., et. al., "Plasma C-reactive protein and homocysteine concentrations are related to frequent fruit and vegetable intake in Hispanic and non-Hispanic white elders." *Journal of Nutrition* 134.4 (2004): 913–918. Print.

Gemma C., et al. "Diets enriched in foods with high antioxidant activity reverse age-induced decreases in cerebella beta-adrenergic function and increases in pro inflammatory cytokines." *Journal of Neuroscience* 22.14 (2002): 6114–6120. Print.

Giovannucci, E., et al. "A prospective study of dietary fat and risk of prostate cancer." *Journal of the National Cancer Institute* 85.19 (1993): 1571–1579. Print.

Grivennikov, Sergei, I. et al. "Immunity, Inflammation and Cancer." *Cell* 140.6 (2010): 883–889. Print.

Gunter, Marc J., Hoover, Donald R. "Insulin, Insulin-Like Growth Factor-1, and Risk of Breast Cancer." *Journal of the National Cancer Institute* 101.1 (2009): 48–60. Print.

Halliwell, B. "Effect of diet on caner development: is oxidative DNA damage a biomarker?" *Free Radical Biological Medicine* 32.1 (2002): 968–974. Print.

Harmon, Brook E., et al. "Nutrient Composition and Anti-inflammatory Potential of a Prescribed Macrobiotic Diet." *Nutrition and Cancer* 67.6 (2015): 933–940. Print.

Harvard Men's Health Watch. "C-Reactive Protein: A New Marker for Cardiac Risk." *Harvard Health Publications* 6.6 (2002): 4–7. Print.

Herbert, J.R., Hurley, T.H. "The effect of dietary exposure on recurrence and mortality in early stage breast cancer." *Breast Cancer Research and Treatment* 51.1 (1998): 17–28. Print.

Joseph, J.A., et al. "Reversal of age-related declines in neuronal signal transduction, cognitive, and motor behavioral deficients with blueberry, spinach, or strawberry dietary supplementation." *Journal of Neuroscience* 19.18 (1999): 8114–8121. Print.

Joshipura, J.K., Hu, F.B., et al. "The effect of fruit and vegetable intake on risk for coronary heart disease." *Annals of Internal Medicine* 134.12 (2001): 1106–1114. Print.

Kash, Peter M., Lombard, Jay, and Tom Monte. *Freedom from Disease. The Breakthrough Approach to Preventing Cancer, Heart Disease, Alzheimer's and Depression by Controlling Insulin.* New York: St. Martin's Press, 2008. Print.

Keck, A.S., Finely, J.W. "Cruciferous vegetables: cancer protective mechanisms of glucosinolate hydrolysis products and selenium." *Integrative Cancer Therapies* 3.1 (2004): 5–12. Print.

Kelly, C.C., et al. "Low grade chronic inflammation in women with polycystic ovarian syndrome." *Journal of Clinical Endocrinology Metabolism* 86.6 (2001): 2453–2455. Print.

Key, T.J., et al. "Diet, nutrition and the prevention of cancer." *Public Health Nutrition* 7.1A (2004): 187–200. Print.

Laugesen M., Elliot, R. "Ischemic heart disease, Type 1 diabetes, and cow milk A1 beta casein." *New Zealand Medical Journal* 116.1168 (2003): U295. Print.

Lucia, M.S., Torkko, K.C. "Inflammation as a target for prostate cancer chemoprevention: pathological and laboratory rationale." *Journal of Urology* 171.2 Suppl (2004): S30–S34. Print.

Ludwig, D.S. "Diet and development of insulin resistance syndrome." *Asia Pacific Journal of Clinical Nutrition* 12 Suppl (2003): S4. Print.

Malin, A.S., et al. "Intake of fruits, vegetables and selected micronutrients in relation to the risk of breast cancer." *International Journal of Cancer* 105.3 (2003): 413–418. Print.

Maron, D.J. "Flavonoids for reduction of atherosclerotic risk." *Current Atherosclerosis Reports* 6.1 (2004): 73–78. Print.

Martin, David S. "From Omnivore to Vegan: The dietary from omnivore to vegan: The dietary education of Bill Clinton." *CNN* 18 Aug. 2011. Accessed 20 Jan. 2015. http://www.cnn.com/2011/HEALTH/08/18/bill.clinton.diet.vegan/

Mates, J.M., et. al., "Role of reactive oxygen species in apoptosis: implications for cancer therapy." *Internal Journal of Biochemical Cell Biology* 32.2 (2000): 157–170. Print.

McCarty, M.F. "Vegan Proteins may reduce the risk of cancer, obesity, and cardiovascular disease by promoting increased glucogon activity." *Medical Hypotheses* 53.6 (1999): 459–485. Print.

McDougall, John, *McDougall Program for Maximum Weight Loss*. New York: Plume Books, 1994. Print.

Meydani, M. "The Boyd Orr Lecture: Nutritional Interventions in aging and age-associated disease." *Proceedings of Nutrition Society* 61.2 (2002): 165–171. Print.

Miyoshi, Y., Funahashi, T., et al. "Association of Serum Adiponectin Levels with Breast Cancer Risk." *Clinical Cancer Research* 9.15 (2003): 5699–5704. Print.

Monetini, L., et al. "Bovine beta-casein antibodies in breast- and bottle-fed infants: their relevance in Type 1 diabetes." *Diabetes Metabolism Res Rev* 17.1 (2001): 51–54. Print.

Monetini, L., et al. "Establishment of T cell lines to bovine beta-casein and beta-casein-service epitopes in patients with type 1 diabetes." *Journal of Endocrinology* 176.1 (2003): pM143–150. Print.

Mozaffarian, D., Pischon,T., et al. "Dietary intake of trans fatty acids and systemic inflammation in women." *America Journal of Clinical Nutrition* 79.4 (2004): 606–612. Print.

Murillo, G., et al. "Cruciferous vegetables and cancer prevention." *Journal of Nutrition and Cancer* 41.1–2 (2001): 17–28. Print.

Navab, M., et al. "HDL and the inflammatory response induced by LDL-oxidatized phospholipids." *Atherosclerosis Thrombosis Vascular Biology* 21.4 (2001): 481–488. Print.

Nelson, M. "Pro-inflammatory Diet Linked to Earlier Death." *American Institute for Cancer Research.* 7 Nov. 2013. Accessed 3 Feb. 2015. http://www.aicr.org/press/press-releases/pro-inflammatory-diet-link-earlier-death.html?referrer=https://www.google.com/

Nestle, Marion. *Food Politics: How the Food Industry Influences Nutrition and Health.* Berkeley: University California Press, 2013. Print.

Ngo, T.H., Barnard, R.J., et. al., "Insulin-Like Growth Factor I (IGF-I) and IGF Binding Protein-1 Modulate Prostate Cancer Cell Growth and Apoptosis: Possible Mediators for the Effects of Diet and Exercise on Cancer Cell Survival." *Endocrinology* 144.6 (2011): 2319–2324. Print.

Norwich BioScience Institutes. "New evidence for Epigenetic Effects of Diet on Healthy Aging." *ScienceDaily* 6 Dec. 2012. Accessed Mar. 10, 2015. https://www.sciencedaily.com/releases/2012/12/121206122232.htm

Ornish, D., Brown, S.E., et al. "Can lifestyle changes reverse coronary heart disease? The Lifestyle Heart Trial." *The Lancet* 336.8715 (1990): 624–626. Print.

Ornish, D., Barnard, RJ., et al., "Intensive Lifestyle Changes May Affect the Progression of Prostate Cancer." *Journal of Urology* 174.3 (2005): 1065–1070. Print.

People. "I might not be around if I hadn't become a vegan." *People* 19 Feb. 2016. Accessed 20 Jan. 2015. http://greatideas.people.com/2016/02/19/bill-clinton-vegan-diet-hillary-campaign-nevada/

Phillips, P.A., Segasothy, M. "Vegetarian Diet: panacea for modern lifestyle diseases?" *QJM* 92.9 (1999): 531–544. Print.

Pritikin, Robert. *The Pritikin Principle: The Calorie Density Solution.* Des Moines: Time-Life Books, 2000. Print.

Pritikin, Robert. *The Pritikin Weight Loss Breakthrough.* New York: Dutton Books, 1998. Print.

Renehan, Andrew G., Tyson, M., et al. "Body-mass index and incidence of cancer: a systemic review and meta-analysis of prospective observational studies." *The Lancet* 371.9612 (2008): 569–578. Print.

Reuter, S., Gupta, S.C., et al. "Oxidative stress, inflammation, and cancer: How are they linked?" *Free Radical Biology Medicine* 49.11 (2010): 1603–1616. Print.

Ridker, P.M., et. al. "Comparison of C-reactive protein and low-density lipoprotein cholesterol levels in the prediction of first cardiovascular events." *New England Journal of Medicine* 347:20 (2002): 1557–1565. Print.

Rock, C. L., Demark-Wahnefried, W. "Nutrition and Survival after the Diagnosis of Breast Cancer: A Review of the Evidence." *Journal of Clinical Oncology* 20.15 (2002): 3302–3316. Print.

Saleem, M., et al., "Tea beverage in chemoprevention of prostate cancer: a mini-review." *Journal of Nutrition and Cancer* 47.1 (2003): 13–23. Print.

Samoan, S., et al. "A mixed fruit and vegetable concentrate increases plasma antioxidant vitamins and folate and lowers plasma homocysteine in men." *Journal of Nutrition* 133.7 (2003): 2188–2193. Print.

Sarkar, F.H., et al. "Soy isoflavones and cancer prevention." *Cancer Investigations* 21.5 (2003): 744–757. Print.

Saxe, Gordon A., Rock, Cheryl L., et al. "Diet and risk for breast cancer recurrence and survival." *Breast Cancer Treatment* 53.3 (1999): 241–253. Print.

Schrezenmeir, J., et al. "Milk and diabetes." *Journal of the American College of Nutrition* 19.2 Suppl (2000): 176S–190S. Print.

Seccareccia F., et al. "Vegetable intake and long-term survival among middle aged men in Italy." *Annals of Epidemiology* 13.6 (2003): 424–430. Print.

Sofi, Francesco, et al. "Adherence to Mediterranean diet and health status: meta-analysis." *British Medical Journal* 337.7671 (2008): 673–675. Print.

Stoll, B.A. "Western nutrition and the insulin resistance syndrome: a link to breast cancer." *European Journal of Clinical Nutrition* 53.2 (1999): 83–87. Print.

Tapiero, H., et al. "Polyphenols: do they play a role in the prevention of human pathologies?" *Biomedical Pharmacotherapies* 56.4 (2002): 200–207. Print.

Taschery, Sara. "Inflammation and cancer: Why your diet is important." *The University of Texas MD Anderson Cancer Center* May 2014. Accessed 15 Mar. 2015. https://www.mdanderson.org/publications/focused-on-health/may-2014/inflamation-cancer-diet.html

Tymchuk, Christopher, N., Barnard, R.J., et. al., "Evidence of an Inhibitory Effect of Diet and Exercise on Prostate Cancer Cell Growth." *Journal of Urology* 166.3 (2001): 1185–1189. Print.

Warner, Jennifer. "Broccoli May Help Fight Cancer Growth. Study Shows Compound in Broccoli May Block Defective Gene Linked to Tumor Growth." *WebMD* 11 March 2011. Accessed 11 Apr. 2015. http://www.webmd.com/cancer/news/20110311/brocolli-may-help-fight-cancer-growth

Willett, Walter. *Eat, Drink, and Be Healthy: The Harvard Medical School Guide to Healthy Eating.* New York: Free Press, 2005. Print.

Step Four

Altshuler, L.H., Maher, J.H. Acupuncture: A physician's primer, Part II. *Journal of Oklahoma Medical Association* 96.1 (2003): 13–19. Print.

Becker, Robert O. *Cross Currents: The Perils of Electropollution, the Promise of Electromedicine.* New York: Penguin Random House, 1990. Print.

Brooks, Megan. "Social isolation rivals hypertension as mortality risk factor." *Medscape* 17 Sept. 2013. Accessed 25 Apr. 2015. http://www.medscape.com/viewarticle/811133

Burmeister, Alice, with Tom Monte. *The Touch of Healing. Energizing Body, Mind, and Spirit with the Art of Jin Shin Jyutsu.* New York: Bantam Books, 1997. Print.

Diego, M.A., Field, T., et al. "Aggressive adolescents benefit from massage therapy." *Adolescence* 37.147 (2002): 597–607. Print.

Field, T. "Violence and touch deprivation in adolescents." *Adolescence* 37.148 (2002): 735–749. Print.

Helliwell, J.F., Huang, H. "Comparing the Happiness Effects of Real and On-Line Friends." *PLoS One* 8.9 (2013): e72754. doi: 10.1371/journal.pone.0072754.

Houseman, J., Dorman, S. "The Alameda County Study: A Systemic, Chrono-logical Review." *American Journal of Health Education* 36.5 (2005): 302–308. Print.

Ireland, M., Olson, M. "Massage therapy and therapeutic touch in children: state of the science." *Alternative Therapeutic Health Medicine* 6.5 (2000): 54–63. Print.

Jaremka, Lisa M., et al. "Marital distress prospectively predicts poorer cellular immune function." *Psychoneuronendocrinology* 38.11 (2013): 2713–2719. Print.

National Kidney Foundation. "Stress and Your Kidneys." *National Kidney Foundation* Accesssed 25 Apr. 2015. https://www.kidney.org/atoz/content/Stress_and_your_Kidneys

Pantell, Matthew, et al. "Social Isolation: A Predictor of Mortality Comparable to traditional Clinical Risk Factors." *American Journal of Public Health* 103.11 (2013): 2056–2062. Print.

Peters, R.M. "The effectiveness of therapeutic touch: a meta-analytic review." *Nursing Science Quarterly* 12.1 (1999): 52–61. Print.

Primal, H., et al. "Chronic stress promotes tumor growth and angiogenesis in a mouse model of ovarian carcinoma." *Nature Medicine* 12.8 (2006): 939–944. Print.

Reiche, Edna Maria Vissoci, et al. "Stress, depression, the immune system, and cancer." *The Lancet Oncology* 5.10 (2004): 617–625.

Rosch, Paul J. "Hans Selye: Birth of Stress." *The America Institute of Stress* Accessed Apr. 12 2015. http://www.stress.org/about/hans-selye-birth-of-stress/

Russek, L.G., Schwartz, G.E. "Perceptions of parental caring predict health status in midlife: a 35-year follow-up of the Harvard Mastery of Stress Study." *Psychosomatic Medcine* 59.2 (1997): 144–199. Print.

Sentient Developments. "Social isolation just as bad as smoking," *Sentient Developments* 3 Sept. 2010. Accessed 25 Apr. 2015. http://www.sentientdevelopments.com/2010/09/social-isolation-just-as-bad-as-smoking.html

Spence, J.E., Olson, M.A. "Quantitative research on therapeutic touch. An integrative review of the literature 1985–1995." *Scandinavian Journal of Caring Science* 11.3 (1997): 183–190. Print.

Taggart, Lynne. *The Intention Experiment.* New York: Atria Paperback, 2007. Print.

World Health Organization. "Traditional Medicine." *World Health Organization Fact Sheet Number 134.* Revised May 2003. Accessed 26 Apr. 2015. http://www.who.int/mediacentre/factsheets/2003/fs134/en/

Vaillant, G.E., Mukamal, K. "Successful Aging." *American Journal of Psychiatry* 158.6 (2001): 839–847. Print.

Williams, R.B., Barefoot, J.C., et al., "Prognostic importance of social and economic resources among medically treated patients with angiographically documented coronary artery disease." *Journal of the American Medical Association* 267.4 (1992): 520–524. Print.

Wilkinson, D.S., Knox, P.L., et al. "The clinical effectiveness of healing touch." *Journal of Alternative Complementary Medicine* 8.1 (2002): 33–47. Print.

Wolf, S., Bruhn, John G. *The Power of Clan: The Influence of Relationships on Heart Disease.* Piscataway, New Jersey: Transaction Publishers, 1998. Print.

Step Five

Blair, S.N., Kohl, H.W., et al. "Physical Fitness and all-cause mortality. A prospective study of healthy men and women." *The Journal of the American Medical Association* 262.17 (1989): 2395–2401. Print.

Boyle, S. H., Jackson, W. G., Suarez, E. C. "Hostility, anger, and depression predict increases in C3 over a 10-year period." *Brain, Behavior, and Immunity* 21.6 (2007): 816–823. Print.

Dardik, Irving. *Making Waves: Irving Dardik and His Superwave Principle.* Emmaus, PA: Rodale Press, 2005. Print.

Duncan, J.J., Gordon N.F., et al. "Women walking for health and fitness. How much is enough?" *The Journal of the American Medical Association* 266.23 (1991): 3295–3299. Print.

Jung, C.G. *Memories, Dreams, and Reflections.* New York: Random House Vintage Books, 1963. Print.

Paffenbarger, Ralph S., Hyde, Robert T., et al. "The Association of Changes in Physical Activity Level and Other Lifestyle Characteristics with Morality Among Men." *New England Journal of Medicine* 328.8 (1993): 538–545. Print.

Pennebaker, James. *Opening Up by Writing it Down, Third Edition.* New York: Guilford Press, 2016. Print.

Penninx, B.W., Gurainik, J.M. "Chronically Depressed Mood and Cancer Risk in Older Persons." *Journal of the National Cancer Institute* 90.24 (1998): 1888–1893. Print.

Sieber, W.J., Rodin, J., et al. "Modulation of human killer cell activity by exposure to uncontrollable stress." *Brain, Behavior, and Immunity* 6.2 (1992): 141–156. Print.

Wood, P.D, Terry, R.B., et al. "Metabolism of Substrates: diet, lipoprotein metabolism, and exercise." *Federation Proceedings* 44.2 (1985): 358–363. Print.

Step Six
Benson, Herbert. *The Relaxation Response.* New York: HarperCollins, 1975. Print.

Boyd, Doug. Rolling Thunder: A Personal Exploration into the Secret Healing Powers of an American Indian Medicine Man. New York: Random House, 1974. Print.

Brother Lawrence. *The Practice of the Presence of God: The Wisdom and Teachings of Brother Lawrence.* Brewster, MA: Paraclete Press, 1985. Print.

Byrd, Randolph C. "Positive Therapeutic Effects of Intercessory Prayer in a Coronary Care Unity Population." *Southern Medical Journal* 81.7 (1988): 826–829. Print.

Chopra, Deepak. *How to Know God.* New York: Harmony Books, 2000. Print.

Cousins, Norman. *Anatomy of an Illness as Perceived by the Patient.* New York: W.W. Norton Company, 1979. Print.

Dispenza, Joe. *Breaking the Habit of Being Yourself.* Carlsbad, CA: Hay House, 2012. Print.

Koenig, Harold G. "Religion, Spirituality, and Health: the Research and Clinical Implications." *International Scholarly Research Network Psychiatry* 2012 (2012): Article ID 278730, 33 pages. Print.

Krucoff, Mitchell W., et al. "Percutaneous intervention during unstable coronary syndromes: Monitoring and Actualization of Noetic Training (MANTRA) feasibility pilot." *American Heart Association Journal* 142.5 (2001): 760–769. Print.

University of California, Los Angeles. "Mindfulness Meditation Slows Progression of HIV, Study Suggests." *ScienceDaily* 27 July 2008. Accessed 30 Apr. 2015. https://www.sciencedaily.com/releases/2008/07/ 080724215644.htm

Monte, Tom. "Mona's Victory over Despair." *East West Journal* November 1981. Print.

Peale, Norman V. *The Power of Positive Thinking*. New York: Touchstone, 2003. Print.

Rabin, Roni Caryn. "Ask Well: The Health Benefits of Meditation." *New York Times* 10 November 2015. Accessed 15 Dec. 2015. http://well.blogs.nytimes.com/2015/11/10/ask-well-the-health-benefits-of-meditation/?_r=0

Reynolds, Gretchen. "How Meditation Changes the Brain and Body." *New York Times* 18 February 2016. Accessed Mar. 1 2016. http://well.blogs.nytimes.com/2016/02/18/contemplation-therapy/

Seligman, Martin E.P. *Learned Optimism*. New York: Random House, 2006. Print.

Talbot, Margaret. "The Placebo Prescription." *New York Times* 9 January 2000. Accessed Mar. 12 2015. http://www.nytimes.com/2000/01/09/magazine/the-placebo-prescription.html

University of Los Angeles. UCLA Mindfulness Awareness Research Center. Accessed 12 May 2015. http://marc.ucla.edu/

Williamson, Marianne. *Everyday Grace*. New York: Riverhead Books, 2002. Print.

Wolf, Fred Alan. *Taking the Quantum Leap: The New Physics for Nonscientists*. San Francisco: Harper and Row Publishers, 1981. Print.

Step Seven

Boscia, Ted. "Life purpose buffers bad moods triggered by diversity." *Cornell Chronicle* 3 September 2013. Accessed 15 May 2015. http://www.news.cornell.edu/stories/2013/09/life-purpose-buffers-bad-moods-triggered-diversity

Rush University Medical Center. "Purpose in Life and Alzheimer's." *Rush University Medical Center* Accessed 17 May 2015. https://www.rush.edu/health-wellness/discover-health/purpose-life-and-alzheimers

Briggs, Helen. "Sense of purpose 'adds years to life.'" *BBC News* 14 May 2014. Accessed 18 May 2015. http://www.bbc.com/news/health-27393057

AARP Foundation Experience Corps. *AARP Foundation* Accessed 18 May 2015. http://www.aarp.org/experience-corps/

Fernandez, Elizabeth. "Lifestyle Changes May Lengthen Telomeres, A Measure of Cell Aging." *UCSF* 16 Sept. 2013. Accessed 19 May 2015. https://www.ucsf.edu/news/2013/09/108886/lifestyle-changes-may-lengthen-telomeres-measure-cell-aging

Hershey, Robert D. "The Rise in Death Rate After New Year Is Tied to Will to See 2000." *New York Times* 15 Jan. 2000. Accessed 15 Mar. 2015. http://www.nytimes.com/2000/01/15/nyregion/rise-in-death-rate-after-new-year-is-tied-to-the-will-to-see-2000.html

Hill, P., Turiano, N.A. "Purpose in Life as a Predictor of Mortality Across Adulthood." *Psychological Science* 25.7 (2014): 1482–1486. Print.

Monte, Tom. *The Way of Hope.* New York: Warner Books, 1990. Print.

Norton, Amy. "How Having a Sense of Purpose Can Help You Stay Healthy." *HealthDay News* 3 Nov. 2014. Accessed 21 May 2015. http://news.health.com/2014/11/04/purpose-in-life-a-boon-to-your-health/

O'Reilly, Dermot, et. al. "Caregiving reduces mortality risk for most caregivers: a census-based record linkage study." *International Journal of Epidemiology* 44.6 (2015): 1959–1969. Print.

Simonton, O. Carl. *Getting Well Again.* New York: Bantam Books, 1980. Print.

Van Ness, Derick. "Find Your Passion: Simple Steps to Discover Who You Are, How to Choose a Career, and How to Find Your Purpose in Life! 2nd Edition" Derick Van Ness, 2013.

The Healing Miracles Within

Taggart, Lynne. *The Intention Experiment.* New York: Atria Paperback, 2007. Print.

World Health Organization. "Traditional Medicine." *World Health Organization Fact Sheet Number 134* Revised May 2003. Accessed 21 May 2015. http://www.who.int/mediacentre/factsheets/2003/fs134/en/

Becker, Robert O. *Cross Currents: The Perils of Electropollution, the Promise of Electromedicine.* New York: Penguin Random House, 1990. Print.

Sattilaro, A., Monte, T. "Physician Heal Thyself. A doctor's remarkable from cancer and the diet he's convinced was responsible." *Life Magazine* August 1982: 62. Print.

Sattilaro, Anthony, with Tom Monte. *Recalled by Life*. Boston: Houghton Mifflin, 1982. Print.

Kohler, Jean. *Healing Miracles from Macrobiotics*. New York: Prentice Hall, 1981. Print.

Exploring the Possibilities
Van Lommel, Pim, et al. "Near-death experience in survivors of cardiac arrest: a prospective study in the Netherlands." *The Lancet* 358.9298 (2001): 2039–2045. Print.

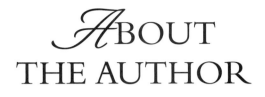

ABOUT THE AUTHOR

Tom Monte has written or coauthored more than thirty-five books on the subjects of health, healing, and personal transformation, including *Freedom from Disease; Taking Woodstock: A True Story of a Riot, Concert, and a Life; The Way of Hope; Recalled by Life;* and *Living Well Naturally.* He has also written hundreds of articles that have appeared in countless leading magazines and newspapers, including the *Saturday Evening Post; the Chicago Tribune; Life; Runner's World;* and *Natural Health.*

Tom has lectured and conducted extended workshops for health, healing, intimate relationships, and personal development throughout the United States and Europe. He is the creator and primary teacher of the Healer's Program, a training program for professional healers; and Living in Alignment, a multi-module program for personal transformation.

You can find out more about Tom Monte at TomMonte.com.

INDEX

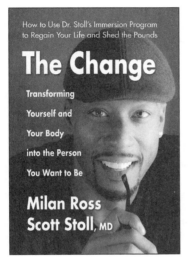

THE CHANGE

Transforming Yourself and Your Body into the Person You Want to Be

Milan Ross and Scott Stoll, MD

Not just another weight-loss book, *The Change* is the true story of how Milan Ross—with the help of Dr. Scott Stoll's unique seven-day immersion program—lost 275 pounds of excess weight and regained control of his life. The book includes not only Milan's day-to-day account of what he accomplished during that crucial week but also the voice of Dr. Stoll, who takes you through the very same program Milan experienced. *The Change* shows you how to lose weight and be healthy not for just a month or a year but for a lifetime.

$24.95 • 240 pages • 6 x 9-inch paperback • ISBN 978-0-7570-0432-2

THE CHANGE COOKBOOK

Using the Power of Food to Transform Your Body, Your Health, and Your Life

Milan Ross and Scott Stoll, MD

From the authors of *The Change* comes a new cookbook based on Dr. Stoll's Immersion program for weight loss and better health. Imagine dishes that can reduce your cholesterol, lower your blood pressure, boost your immune system, and decrease your odds of suffering from cancer, type 2 diabetes, heart disease, stroke, or a host of other all-too-common health problems. Here, in this new book, are over 150 recipes that can truly change your life for the better.

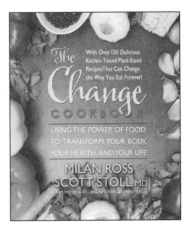

$17.95 • 256 pages • 7.5 x 9-inch paperback • ISBN 978-0-7570-0438-4

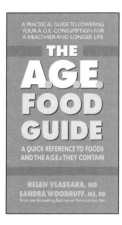

THE AGE FOOD GUIDE
A Quick Reference to Foods and the AGEs They Contain
Helen Vlassara, MD and Sandra Woodruff, RD

All foods contain naturally occurring toxic substances called AGEs—advanced glycation end products. Studies have shown that a buildup of AGEs increases oxidation and free radicals, hardens tissue, and creates chronic inflammation, leading to a host of illnesses. While many foods contain high AGE levels, many others contain very little. By knowing the best foods to choose and their optimal preparation methods, you can lower your consumption of these harmful substances. *The AGE Food Guide* is designed to help. This comprehensive guide lists hundreds of common foods and their AGE levels. In an easy-to-follow format, the foods are listed both alphabetically and within categories for quick and easy access.

With *The AGE Food Guide* in hand, you can confidently make wise food choices that will allow you to enjoy greater health and longevity.

$8.95 • 224 pages • 4 x 7-inch paperback • ISBN 978-0-7570-0429-2

DR. VLASSARA'S A.G.E.-LESS DIET
How Chemicals in the Foods We Eat Promote Disease, Obesity, and Aging And the Steps We Can Take to Stop It
Helen Vlassara, MD, Sandra Woodruff, MS, RD, Gary E. Striker, MD

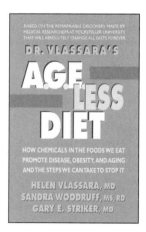

Imagine naturally occurring substances that are responsible for chronic disease and accelerated aging. When trying to discover why diabetes patients were prone to complications such as heart disease, Helen Vlassara and her research team focused on compounds called *advanced glycation end products,* or *AGEs,* which enter the body through the diet. For years, these amazing studies remained unknown to the public. Now, Dr. Vlassara, Dr. Gary Striker, and best-selling author Sandra Woodruff have written a complete guide to understanding what AGEs are and how to avoid them through the careful selection of foods and cooking techniques.

$16.95 • 328 pages • 6 x 9-inch paperback • ISBN 978-0-7570-0420-9

THE BOOK OF MACROBIOTICS

The Universal Way of Health, Happiness & Peace

Michio Kushi with Alex Jack

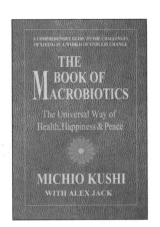

The Book of Macrobiotics is a passport to a world of understanding. It has been studied by hundreds of thousands of people in search of a comprehensive approach to living in a world of constant change.

Now, after two decades, this classic has been revised and expanded to reflect refinements in Michio Kushi's teachings, as well as developments in the modern practice of macrobiotics. The standard macrobiotic diet has been simplified and broadened, and macrobiotic approaches to cancer, heart disease, and other disorders have evolved and expanded, as have basic home care and lifestyle recommendations.

$17.95 • 432 pages • 6 x 9-inch paperback • ISBN 978-0-7570-0342-4

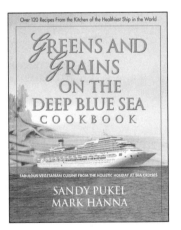

GREENS AND GRAINS ON THE DEEP BLUE SEA COOKBOOK

Fabulous Vegetarian Cuisine from the Holistic Holiday at Sea Cruises

Sandy Pukel and Mark Hanna

You are invited to come aboard one of America's premier health cruises. Too busy to get away? Even if you can't swim in the ship's pool, you can still enjoy its gourmet cuisine, because natural foods expert Sandy Pukel and master chef Mark Hanna have created *Greens & Grains on the Deep Blue Sea Cookbook*—a titanic collection of the most popular vegetarian dishes served aboard the Holistic Holiday at Sea cruises.

Each of the book's more than 120 recipes is designed to provide not only great taste, but also maximum nutrition. Choose from among an innovative selection of taste-tempting appetizers, soups, salads, entrées, side dishes, and desserts. Easy-to-follow instructions ensure that even novices have superb results. With *Greens & Grains on the Deep Blue Sea Cookbook,* you can enjoy fabulous signature dishes from the Holistic Holiday at Sea cruises in the comfort of your own home.

$16.95 • 160 pages • 7.5 x 9-inch paperback • ISBN 978-0-7570-0287-8

VICKI'S VEGAN KITCHEN

Eating with Sanity, Compassion & Taste

Vicki Chelf

Vegan dishes are healthy and delicious, yet many people are daunted by the idea of preparing meals that contain no animal products. For them, and for everyone who loves great food, vegetarian chef Vicki Chelf presents a comprehensive cookbook designed to take the mystery out of meatless meals. The book begins with an overview of the vegan diet and chapters on kitchen staples, cooking methods, and food preparation. Over 375 of Vicki's favorite recipes follow—and each one is easy to make and utterly delectable.

$17.95 • 320 pages • 7.5 x 9-inch paperback • ISBN 978-0-7570-0251-9

GOING WILD IN THE KITCHEN

The Fresh & Sassy Tastes of Vegetarian Cooking

Leslie Cerier

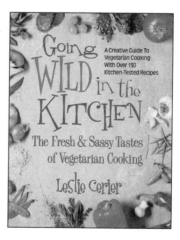

Venture beyond the usual beans, grains, and vegetables to include an exciting variety of organic vegetarian fare in your meals. *Going Wild in the Kitchen* shows you how. Author Leslie Cerier offers over 150 kitchen-tested recipes for taste-tempting dishes that contain such unique ingredients as edible flowers; wild mushrooms, berries, and herbs; and exotic ancient grains like teff, quinoa, and Chinese "forbidden" black rice. Leslie also encourages your creative instincts by prompting you to "go wild" and add new ingredients to existing recipes.

$16.95 • 240 pages • 7.5 x 9-inch paperback • ISBN 978-0-7570-0091-1

For more information about our books, visit our website at www.squareonepublishers.com